contents *book*

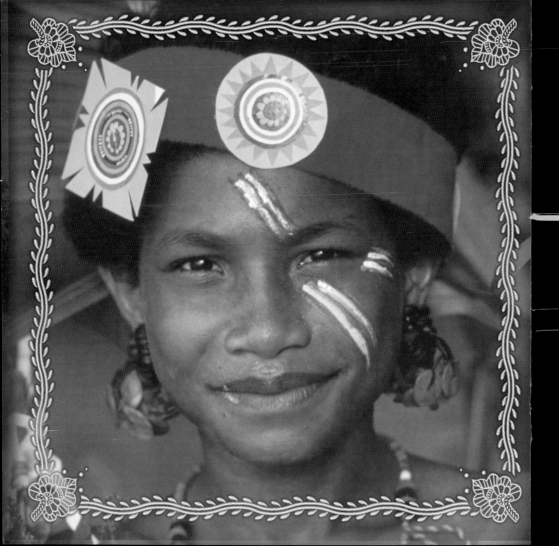

INTRODUCTION

Decorated skin—a celebration of the body and mind performed by our civilizations past and present—is a truly expressive example of the human spirit in action.

We are incredibly conscious of our outward appearance and are aware that our skin can provide a rich backdrop for human self-expression. Body painting, tattooing, piercing, and scarification are used all over the world as a way of marking special moments in our lives. The human body can be transformed and reshaped, turned into a living canvas of color and markings, signifying pain and sorrow, spiritual belief, joy, endurance, and cultural identity.

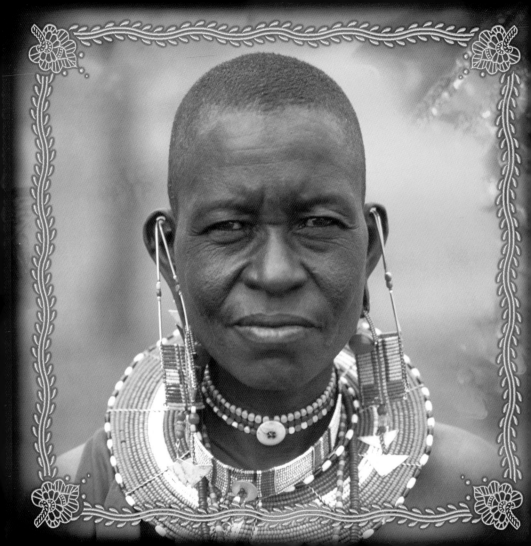

Ancient rituals are continually being discovered, formed and molded by time and evolve into tribal custom. As new unearthing of the past continues, we are increasingly amazed at our ancestors' diverse way of life, and the many interesting methods they used to prove their worth within their community.

Some chose scarification for ethnic identity; shaping their scars into circles and shapes to show their respect for tribal customs. Some preferred painting their bodies, using different types of clay and henna. Many developed tattooing into a permanent art form, while other cultures pierced themselves on the face with sharp objects, and inserted bones to appear fearsome to their enemies.

Contemporary body art is an ever-changing craft. As the world of information has opened up and become easily available to all, our own generation has transformed body art. The shock level experienced when the Punk culture introduced excessive body piercing has diminished somewhat, although many still find some of the piercings and ornaments worn today quite unacceptable. Eyebrows, lips, tongues, and other parts of the body can all be perforated, but the majority of us prefer less outrageous decoration, settling for simple ear or nose jewelry.

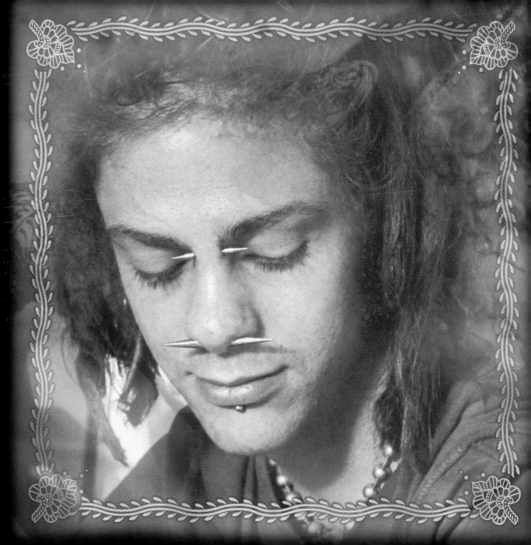

Body art has many other forms. People readily choose to be tattooed, selecting patterns at will and sometimes eventually covering much of their bodies with colorful scenes and symbols.

Many of the most popular designs are based on ancient motifs as we continue our quest to emulate the past. The method of introducing color into the skin with a sharp implement has remained similar for generations, and tattooing has developed into a modern expression of history. Alongside the permanency of tattooing is the use of colored body paints. An equally effective tool of the body art trade are body paints, which wash off with water and are far less messy than mankind's earliest paint, mud!

Most forms of body art can be either temporary or permanent, and the many ways in which people can change, modify, decorate, and adorn their bodies are endless. It can be a painful process, but the pain is considered to be a rite of passage for some, a testimony to their inner strength and courage.

Our modern world is less concerned with ethnic identity, instead preferring to enhance our own uniqueness in an attempt to be noticed. We all have our own concept of beauty and, across the great cultural divide, the desire to transform the body into our preferred appearance knows no boundaries.

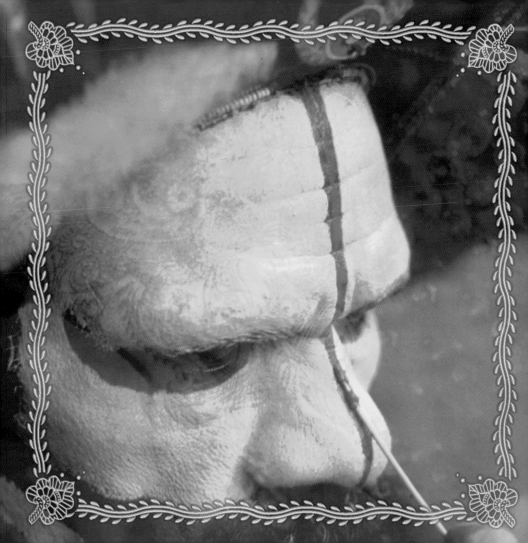

PAIN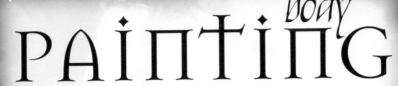TING

In our fast-paced, modern world, it is easy to forget that many of our contemporary practices originated from our past.

Body painting for the purposes of advertising and decoration is common today, with many different types of ready-made paints and substances easily available to everyone.

Painting the body was common practice for some of our ancestors. They used this art form as a way of marking special events and invoking spiritual awareness of people and their surroundings.

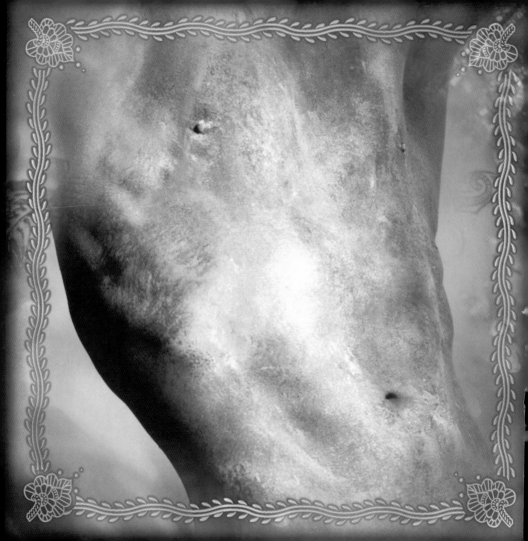

Australasia, the Far East, the Middle East, Europe, and the Americas—every country in the world has a long tradition of body painting. Different substances and patterns abound, but the traditional purpose remains the same—the temporary decoration of the body for specific moments of spiritual connection.

The special tradition of using different designs and colors on the body to tell a story is still as important a ritual today as it was thousands of years ago.

A Natural Canvas

Modern artists use the body as a canvas to establish corporate identities and to promote anything from beer to chocolate, music to magazines. Painting a naked body to appear clothed is the latest craze sweeping the advertising and modeling world. The illusion that the body is clothed can be absolutely complete, with most onlookers not aware that the person is wearing nothing but paint.

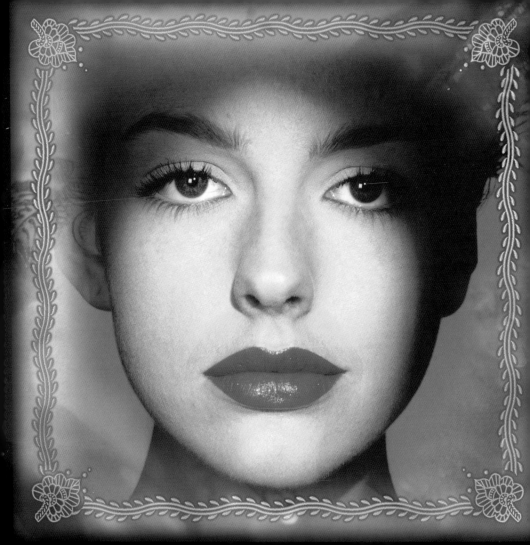

Body paint is generally easy to apply and remove, and is probably the most temporary of all the forms of body art. Painting the body creates a short-term fantasy, which disappears at will, as opposed to tattooing or scarification which mark a person for life.

Contemporary men and women paint their faces in order to appear more attractive—eyelashes, cheeks, lips all enhanced by the temporary application of color. Pale bodies are transformed into tanned masterpieces for that moment on the beach! Even children become someone or something else once face paints are applied—a cat, a superhero, or a pretty flower. And let's not forget sports fans who visually support their team in glorious technicolor from head to toe!

When you change your appearance with body paint, you are an extension of an ancient tradition of body art. For that fleeting moment, you mirror someone else and become part of an ongoing ritual which has been around for centuries.

Traditional Pigments

Many different pigments have been traditionally used to paint the body across the world, each having its own significance. Among the more traditional is ochre, used by Aborigines to invoke a spiritual connection to the land by incorporating the earth into their rituals through painting their bodies.

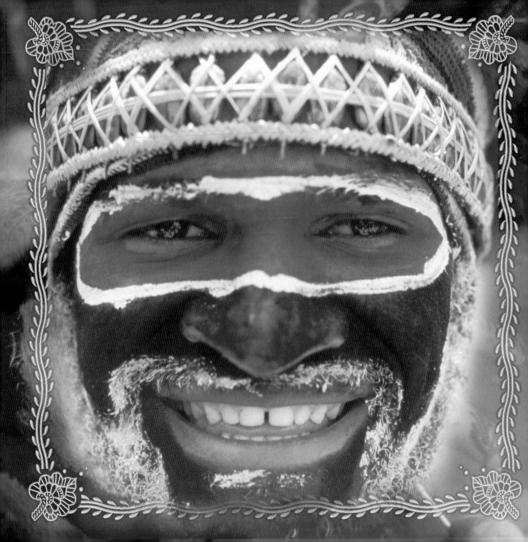

Ochre was traded throughout Asia, Africa and Europe, along with camwood, cinnabar, and kaolin, which is a special body paint formed from white clay. Used for centuries by some African tribes for the protection of a mother and her newborn child, applying kaolin paste is thought to allow healers to communicate with spirits to aid healing of the sick.

Henna's History

Probably the most commonly known and most popular body paint throughout the world today is henna. Although India is traditionally the home of henna body art, it may be surprising to know that this art has also been practiced for thousands of years in Africa and the Middle East. Used to decorate the body for important occasions and celebrations, henna is known to have a cooling effect on the skin.

Henna was widely traded in the Muslim world along with patterns and designs. Derived from *Lawsonia Inermis* and obtained by crushing the dried leaves of the bush, the powder is often mixed with natural ingredients to form a paste.

Henna has been used for centuries by many different cultures and still has an important role to play in contemporary society. Although natural henna is green in color, the stain left on the body once the paste is removed is reddish-brown which will gradually fade. Pure henna is always the safest to use.

17

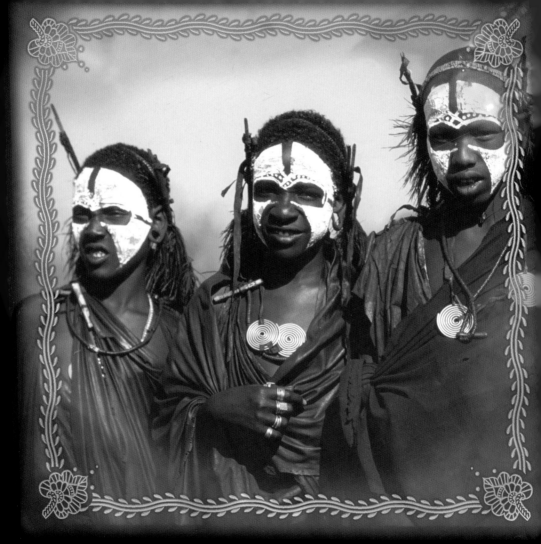

India's Traditions

When you think of henna, the images of beautifully decorated hands and feet come to mind, evocative of the mysterious world of Indian Mehndi. There are many definitions of Mehndi, but it is an all encompassing word that's difficult to explain. It is the cultural art of decorating the body for a special occasion with a paste made from henna powder. The artist, the wearer and the "baraka" or "power over evil" are all brought together when Mehndi is applied.

Although the history of henna in India is not as ancient as many other cultures, somehow it has become a powerful symbol of Indian life. In the early history of Indian henna design, palms and soles were dipped into a fresh paste of crushed leaves known as dip henna, whereas in Middle Eastern henna the paste was applied with a stick.

Ancient Artifacts

Made in about 400 AD, the first artifacts depicting hennaed hands in India were found in the Ajanta caves. Also in the caves are paintings of men and women of all classes, deities and demons each with hennaed hands and feet.

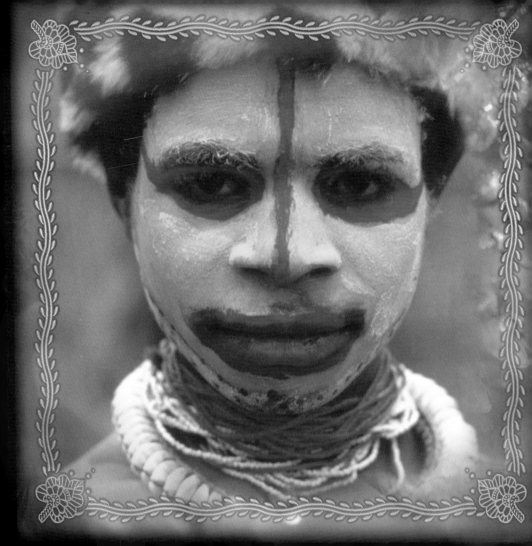

In paintings and sculptures from 600 AD to 1300 AD found in northern India and bordering countries, solid bright red palms and soles appear on humans, demons, clerics and even Buddha himself. To this day, Hindu deities are still shown with red palms and soles.

Miniature paintings during that time show women with red tinted hands and feet, but the henna is still seen as a fairly solid block of color and not patterned. The Persian women glimpsed in the early Mogul courts of India wore ornate black henna patterning on their skin but this did not have any effect on the Indian Mehndi style.

Mehndi Style

Dip henna was common in India until around 1500 BC and patterning remained very simple for at least 100 years after that. Most women portrayed by Indian artists are still depicted with red dip henna and simple patterning.

By the 19th century, complex, elaborate Mehndi had became an established tradition in Hindu India, used by women to enhance their beauty. Today, it is usually applied for the celebration of weddings and holidays.

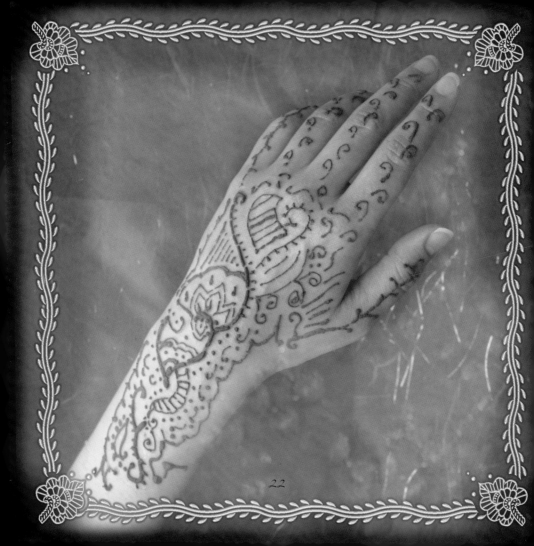

22

South Indian classical dancers have a special design which was used by Asian elders. Simple to apply, a circular pattern, which is filled in, is drawn in the center of the palm of the hand. Then a cap is formed on the fingertips by dipping them in Mehndi.

Mehndi and Marriage

The "Night of the Henna," the Mehndi ritual preparing the bride for marriage was well established among Muslims by 1700 AD. Indian brides have the most intricate and intense patterns applied to their bodies, and during the hours it takes to fix the dye, they are regaled with good advice about the wedding night by their giggling friends.

Traditionally, the groom's name is hidden in the design and he may not consummate the marriage until he has found his name on her palm, although this is also seen as a ruse to let him touch her hands and thus initiate a physical relationship. If he fails to find his name, however, it is said that the bride will become more dominant during their marriage.

The bride is held in such high esteem that until the henna fades, she is excused from any housework. Another tradition in Northern India is that the longer the henna lasts, the longer the love will last between the lucky couple.

23

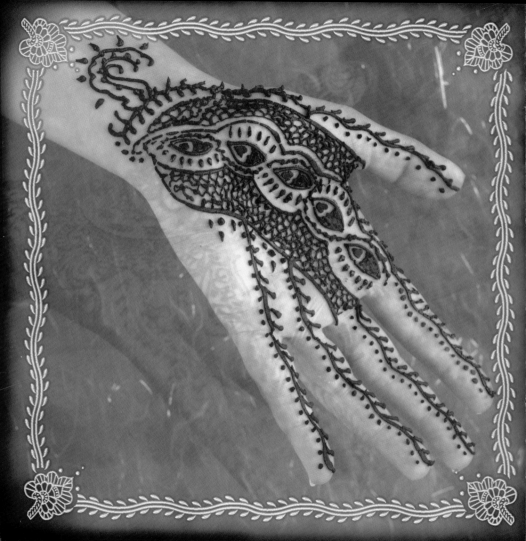

Women and Henna

Henna painting is customarily considered a female art form, used as a marker of special events during a woman's lifetime. As she passes through each phase of her life, such as puberty, marriage and childbirth, she will be decorated with henna to ensure her ongoing good fortune. Although the henna is sometimes used as a form of jewelry, it is traditionally associated with transcendence and transformation, and is not applied simply for pleasure or vanity.

Once a woman is married, Mehndi becomes a festive expression of her special position in her family and her deep-rooted devotion to loved ones. She becomes strong enough to save the family from disaster and even her celebratory prayers are for the welfare of her family. In Indian society her worth is recognized and revered and she will wear her henna proudly as a symbol of her status.

Hindu Rituals with Henna

The Indian Hindu people also have a deep bond with henna adornment. Henna is a great hair conditioning dye and is used by both men and women. Feasts and fasts are occasions for henna application and even gods and goddesses are depicted with Mehndi designs drawn on their bodies.

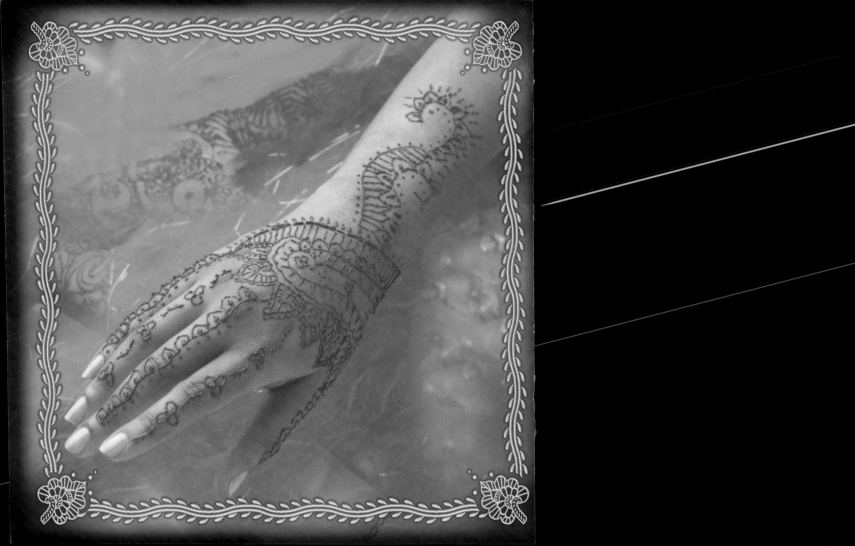

A Hindu bride-to-be goes through the Mehndi ritual the day before her wedding. She gathers her friends together and decorates their hands, wrists, palms, and feet with henna, and they in turn paint her. The Hindu marriage is a very special time and the ornaments drawn on the bride's body have great significance.

Many of the religious rites before, and during, a Hindu wedding include henna, and marriage would be considered incomplete if these rituals were ignored. The reddish-brown color stands for the affluence a bride is expected to bring her new family while the deeper the color and the longer the dye lasts delays her return to housework.

Unmarried friends are not left out of the excitement. Just as we try to catch the Western bride's bouquet, they receive scrapings of Mehndi leaves from the bride which are considered lucky and may lead the unmarried to a suitable marital match.

Celebration and Healing

The traditions of Mehndi cross the boundaries of all Indian culture and its uses are established and revered. It is used for celebration and to mark auspicious occasions. Many Indians would consider it a vital part of their tribal and traditional customs, their special moments remembered forever by a design of beauty upon their skin.

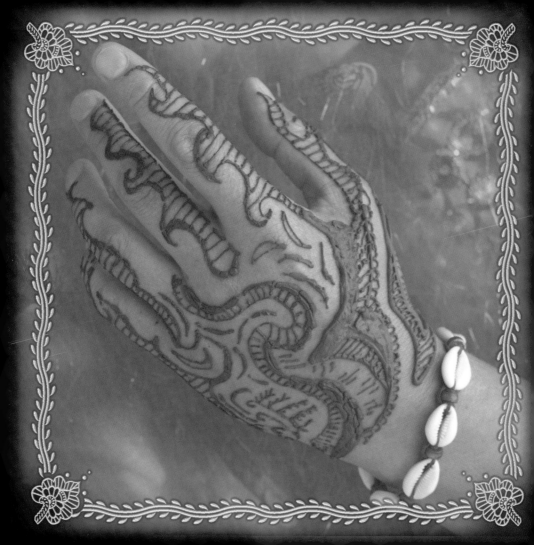

Henna in North Africa

In ancient times, henna was used throughout North Africa for its remarkable healing properties when applied to the skin. Cuts and bruises, many skin disorders, headaches, and fevers were all helped by its medicinal content. It is not known exactly when Mehndi began to evolve but certainly the people of North Africa have an age-old tradition of using henna patterns, confined mainly to the hands and feet. The style generally follows the shape of the feet and the hands incorporate geometrical floral patterns.

Among North African women, there is a strong traditional belief in the power of symbols used to promote protection and fertility. The evil eye is seen by all as being responsible for any misfortune and many of the popular designs are used in the hope of deflecting its malevolence elsewhere.

The Berbers use a popular emblem in their designs, a cross at the center of two diamonds. Diamonds supposedly ward off the evil eye and one inside the other with a cross in the center is seen as powerful enough to send the evil energy in four different directions.

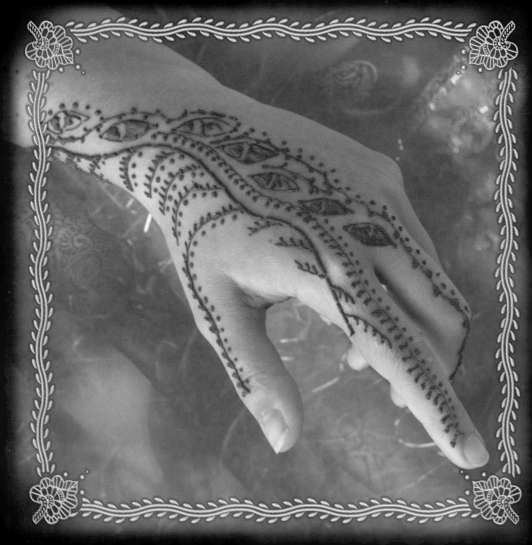

Geometric shapes such as triangles, crosses, circles, and spirals are commonly seen as having varied symbolic meanings. The most popular patterns include geometric, floral designs and borders with bold patterns. A young girl in puberty may bear palm branch designs to enhance her childbearing potential. The serpent, which represents a royal emblem in Africa, has great significance—it can denote immortality or protection of the earth, among other interpretations. It may only be worn by those deemed worthy of the honor.

To the Sudanese people, henna has a special meaning of happiness. By wearing henna, a wife shows her love for her husband—by not putting it on her body, she indicates a lack of affection for him. As in other North African cultures, a wife will not wear henna after her husband's death.

Moroccan Mehndi

Moroccan women use Mehndi patterns to protect them from evil, and to promote luck and fertility. Henna is regarded as having "baraka" (blessing) and has the power to dispel "djinn" (evil spirits), that can cause diseases and sterility.

An interesting tradition, continued by the Moroccan women of today, is the holding of a three-day event during which dancers use

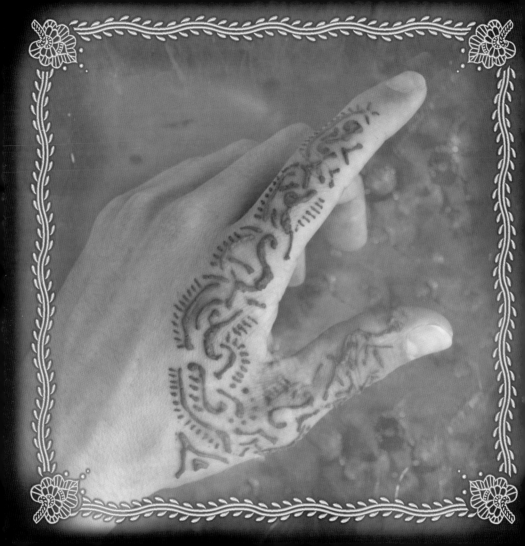

Mehndi and jewelry to draw attention to their hands and feet. In one of the dances, called the "Guedra" (Dance of Love), specific patterns are designed to attract a man's eye to the sinuous movement of the dancer's fingers.

There are many symbolic moments in a woman's life which involve henna, including her wedding day when her hair is coated with henna paste, her first visit to her in-laws seven months after the wedding, and a second visit a year later, when a symbol of stability is drawn in her palm.

During her seventh month of pregnancy, she may visit a henna artist. To protect both her and her unborn child until after the birth, a woman's ankle is decorated with a symbol repeated on an amulet applied at the same time.

Moroccan men have prenuptial henna parties. The groom goes through a ritual of applying a special concoction of henna paste to his hands. His friends then dance around the room taking turns to balance a bowl with lit candles on their heads. When the bowl breaks, the event is over.

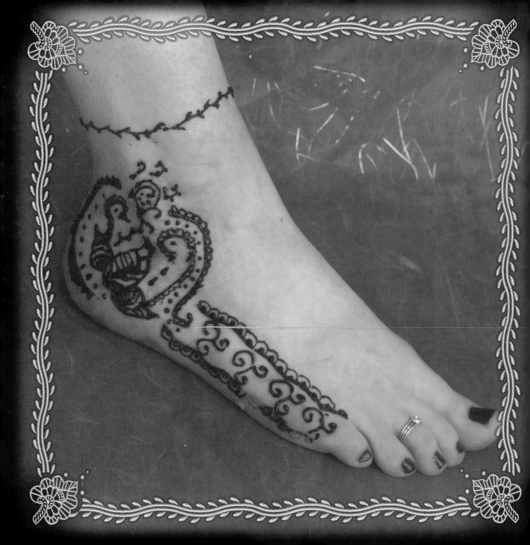

Symbolism of the Body

As already seen, the henna plant is thought to be spiritually powerful, and Mehndi patterns are used to protect the user from evil spirits entering the body, especially around the eyes. Mehndi designs are also applied to a woman's face, hands, and feet to protect her, especially during transitional stages in her life that are considered to be her most dangerous times—puberty, marriage, pregnancy, birth, and death.

A woman may apply henna to the palm of her husband's hand to protect him as he goes to war.

If widowed, she may not wear henna for four months after his death.

At his funeral a male will have henna scattered on his head and mourners will often dip their hands in henna to soothe their emotions. To encourage joy in her next life, Mehndi is painted on the hands and feet of a woman in death so the link continues.

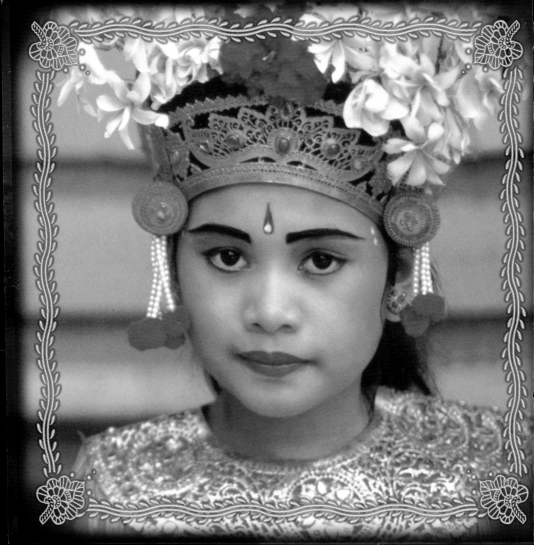

Middle Eastern Traditions

The true origin of henna use in the Middle East is not defined but the many people of the region have used it for thousands of years.

Goddesses of fertility and the battlefield, and the bull god are depicted on shrine walls at Catal Huyuk dated 7000 BC, all with red hands patterned with ornamental designs.

This religion was the precursor to the Bronze Age Middle Eastern religions, which used henna in their fertility rites to worship different goddesses. It is possible that female henna traditions have been practiced since that time, with many artifacts showing fertility goddesses with hennaed hands.

Female statuettes from the Cylacdic Islands, dated around 3500 BC, have red pigment on their hands, as do statuettes from Babylon from

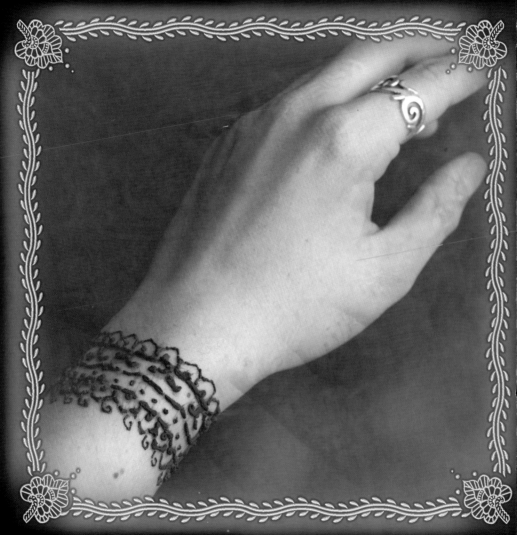

around 2100 BC, both possibly indicating the use of henna at this time. The epic poem of Baal and Anath, also dated around 2100 BC, is the earliest written record of bridal and fertility henna festivals. It implied the use of henna by the Canaanite people as a bridal tradition and a woman's celebration of life; the bride decorating her hands with henna before meeting her husband at a spring fertility festival.

Many more statues made from around 1700 BC to 1 AD show similar examples of henna markings on their hands. Sometimes, the breast and feet also show henna-stained patterns. Minoa, Mycenae, Libya, Iraq, Palestine, Greece, Egypt, Crete, Sicily, Sardinia, Minorca, and Rome—artifacts from these areas depict women with henna patterns on their hands and sometimes on the palms and the soles of their feet. The use of henna was obviously widespread across the region.

From the earliest historical period recorded, henna has been used in Palestine and is mentioned in the Bible as "camphire" in the Song of Solomon. The Romans recorded Gentile and Jewish henna use and an Assyrian text from 800 BC describes a bride being hennaed in preparation for her wedding.

Evidence in Egypt

We know that the art of Mehndi has existed for centuries, although there are many schools of thought about its origination in the Middle East. It was discovered that, as long ago as 1200 BC, henna was painted on the fingers and toes of Pharaohs before the mummification process began, in the hope of pleasing the god and to ensure acceptance into the afterlife. Higher born Egyptian woman also used henna to color their hair and fingernails.

There are some extremely symbolic henna designs which have deep meaning for Egyptians, such as the Moon and the Sun.

Everyday traditional patterns drawn for pleasure include the zigzag or wavy line, the lotus motif and the spiral, said to signify the wonderings of the soul.

Arabia and Beyond

Henna traditions were long established in Arabia, but it is said that the men and women of the Muslim faith began using henna to color their hair and beards around 632 BC, following the reported practice of the prophet Muhammad, who also dyed his beard with henna.

As Islam expanded into other countries, the use of henna spread all over the Middle East and parts of Europe. Grown and used in Spain by Christians, Jews, and Moors, henna became very popular as its properties were shared with Europe.

Muslims all over the world still celebrate the "Night of the Henna" and consider henna a beautiful female ornament.

There are some interesting recorded uses of henna by the Bedouins, who lived near Kuwait one hundred years ago. The women mainly used henna to draw traditional designs on their hands. Many of the men were pearl divers so they used henna on their hands and feet to toughen up the skin for their aquatic adventures.

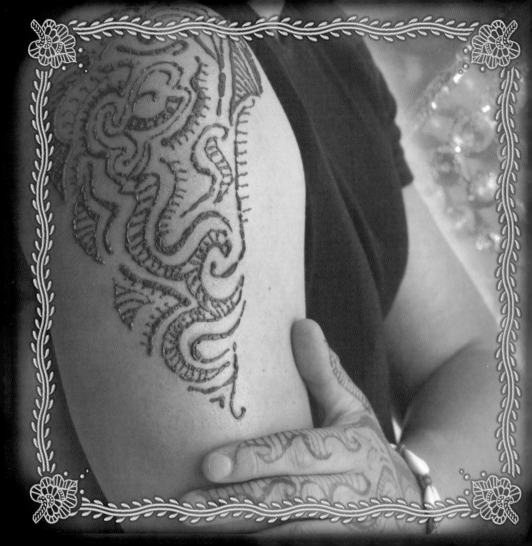

Traditional Iranian henna art has been passed down from generation to generation by henna artists of great repute. It is described as elaborate and ornate and the designs are very complex. Artifacts and texts from as early as 2000 BC demonstrate the origins of henna traditions in Iran which are still a part of the country's lifestyle today.

The Middle Eastern style of Mehndi is mostly made up of floral patterns similar to Arabic textiles, paintings and carvings. In general, simpler patterns such as a solid colored palm or sole are used for everyday wear and more intricate patterns for special occasions, such as weddings and feast days. Sometimes the nails are dyed red to match the designs which are often built up around a central design allowing plenty of skin to be seen as well.

The use of Mehndi for weddings is still crucial. The decorating of the bride's feet and hands is done with much excitement and celebration before her wedding. It is rather sad that some henna traditions have faded in the modern world as Middle Eastern women want to be more like their Western cousins. Fortunately, those same Western cousins have discovered the beauty of henna and so perhaps the wheel will turn back on itself again.

Henna in Southeast Asia

Henna is used in Southeast Asia mainly among the Muslim cultures found there. The importance of henna, during marriage rites, is a crucial moment for the success of the marriage, as we have seen elsewhere.

It is considered a good omen for the bride if the stain lasts a long time, for it is said the longer it remains, the more the bride's new mother-in-law will love her. The merrymaking and rejoicing at the traditional "Night of the Henna" before the marriage is a very exciting time for all involved.

An ancient language of symbols, true Mehndi is a combination of intricate designs with special meaning for the wearer.

There are many common motifs such as flowers for joy, leaves for the harvest, mandalas (which are circles), and bundakis (small dots that represent falling rain.)

Sri Lankan designs are fine and lacy with a paisley pattern, very delicate and pretty. In other regions, sometimes the fingers and toe tips are completely covered in henna. Other designs are similar to the Indian patterns and can be quite plain. The reddish color is considered very beautiful and the bringer of good luck and is used to celebrate marriage, holidays, and family events.

Each community has created its own unique designs, inspired by the surrounding environment, beliefs and religious traditions. Wherever you go in Southeast Asia you are sure to come across women showing off their beautiful hennaed hands.

Indonesia and the Philippines

Long associated with the art of henna, Indonesia and the Philippines continue the tradition today. Henna artists can be found everywhere and are very popular with tourists.

Unfortunately, along with many artists in Europe, they are associated with the latest fashion of using "black" henna to complete their designs which has certain health risks (see page 48). If you do decide to have a henna design from a street artist, it is best to make sure that the henna is untainted.

Body Painting and Henna in the West

As we know, henna has been used for body painting for centuries and Europe is no exception. There is evidence suggesting that henna was used in the Greek Islands around 1700 BC. As their culture developed, the physical appearance of the upper class was enhanced by many artificial aids.

Around 1000 BC, Ancient Greek women apparently spread henna on their hands to make them look younger and both men and women wore wigs to hide their hair, which was seldom washed.

*Because of their worship
of the goddess Hecate,
Greek women stained their feet and hands
with henna, its red color associated
with their own lifegiving blood.*

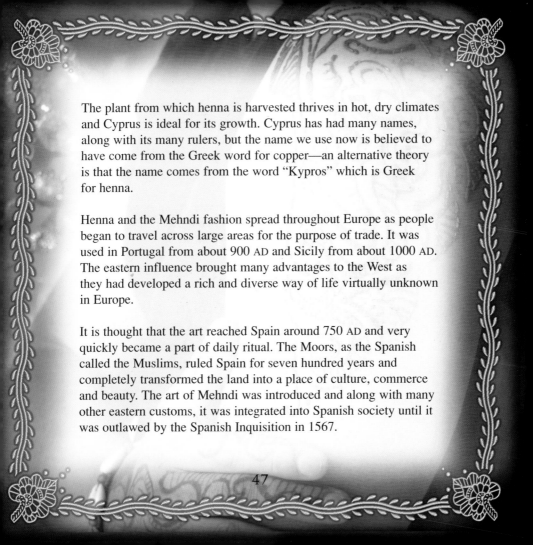

The plant from which henna is harvested thrives in hot, dry climates and Cyprus is ideal for its growth. Cyprus has had many names, along with its many rulers, but the name we use now is believed to have come from the Greek word for copper—an alternative theory is that the name comes from the word "Kypros" which is Greek for henna.

Henna and the Mehndi fashion spread throughout Europe as people began to travel across large areas for the purpose of trade. It was used in Portugal from about 900 AD and Sicily from about 1000 AD. The eastern influence brought many advantages to the West as they had developed a rich and diverse way of life virtually unknown in Europe.

It is thought that the art reached Spain around 750 AD and very quickly became a part of daily ritual. The Moors, as the Spanish called the Muslims, ruled Spain for seven hundred years and completely transformed the land into a place of culture, commerce and beauty. The art of Mehndi was introduced and along with many other eastern customs, it was integrated into Spanish society until it was outlawed by the Spanish Inquisition in 1567.

It is perhaps symbolic of our Western world that we have adopted, and made fashionable, a traditional custom used for the adornment of the poorest women of the East. Unable to afford jewelry, they painstakingly created beautiful designs on their hands and feet. These very same designs have become very desirable to some of the richest women in the world who delight in replicating the mystery of the East.

The temporary, and painless, properties surrounding Mehndi have made the process all the more attractive. Although very much a toy of the rich and famous, the deep and spiritual meanings, which are such an integral part of the Mehndi, are being absorbed by the patrons of this art.

Black Henna—A Word of Warning

The spread of this wonderful Eastern custom throughout Western Europe and much of our modern world has been phenomenal. Unfortunately though, as with all good things, there are risks attached to sharing the Mehndi experience. In a desire to accommodate our demand for stronger color, a new form of henna called "Black Henna" has emerged.

Freely available and used by many artists, black henna is now being highlighted as a dangerous substance. The henna is mixed with a toxic dye, para-phenylenediamine or PPD, which speeds up the dyeing process and results in very black paste. The dye is absorbed by the skin and, unlike pure henna, can cause long-term scarring to the skin and damage to internal organs. Pure henna will normally result in a dark or red brown stain on the skin and the thick, spinachy and earthy smell of real henna is unmistakable.

Natural Designs for the Body

Western men and women choose to paint Mehndi on parts of the body which would never be considered suitable by Eastern culture. The belly button and the back are often adorned—both of which would be forbidden to traditional wearers.

The more subtle designs and symbols are much favored now and have largely replaced the flamboyant tattoos worn by celebrities. It is much easier to have a henna design applied and less of a commitment since it will only last about three weeks.

The fact that henna is completely natural brings its own reward and few allergies to pure henna have been recorded, but it would be wise to heed the earlier warning about the use of unnatural henna. It is a

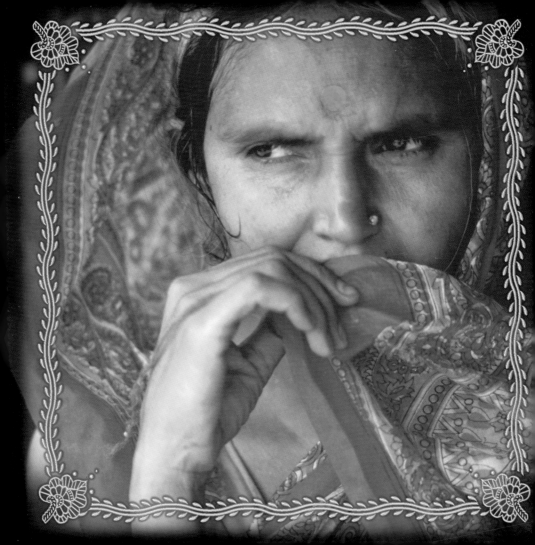

patient craft which cannot be rushed. The longer the henna is left on the skin, the stronger the resulting color and the longer the design will last.

APPLYING YOUR OWN HENNA

The final color of any henna design will be enhanced if the henna is left on for at least 2-8 hours. Initially the henna should be kept damp with a mixture of lemon juice and sugar until the paste turns black. Then the mixture can then be crumbled off when ready. The orange-red color will gradually darken to brown, and if moisturizer is used, the design should last several weeks.

Before using any new supply of henna, perfom a patch test by adding a small amount of the paste to the inside of your arm. Use as instructed and observe the area for 24 hours, if irritation occurs discontinue use.

Designs can either be applied freehand, using the illustrations for inspiration, or with templates. Whatever your design, use it as a means of self expression and celebration.

51

Henna Designs

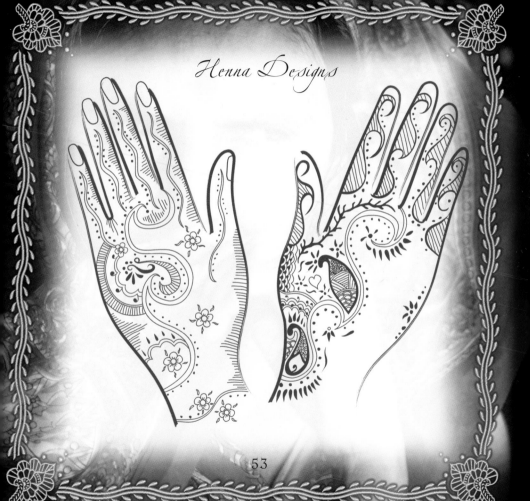

Henna Designs

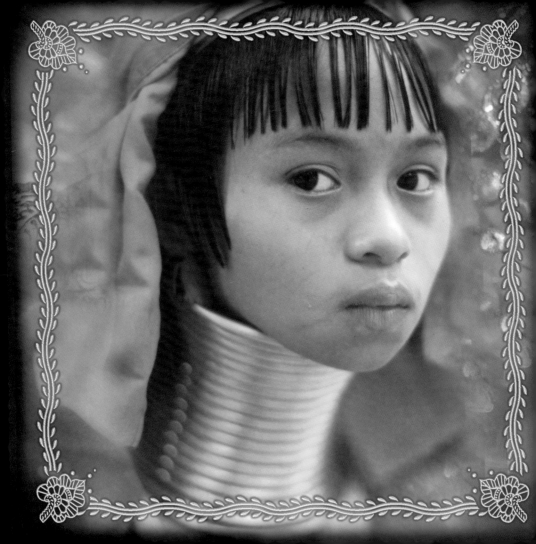

extremes of body ADORNMENT

Shaping, molding and marking bodies
of both men and women of all ages can be very
drastic, and some practices are quite shocking
to our Western culture.
The process is often very painful,
signifying a rite of passage which will
enhance attractiveness.

Changing the shape of the head, the feet, and the waist by
deliberately forcing bodies into altered size or contours, and marking
the skin by cutting it and shaping the subsequent scar, are all part of
the ongoing human quest for perfection.

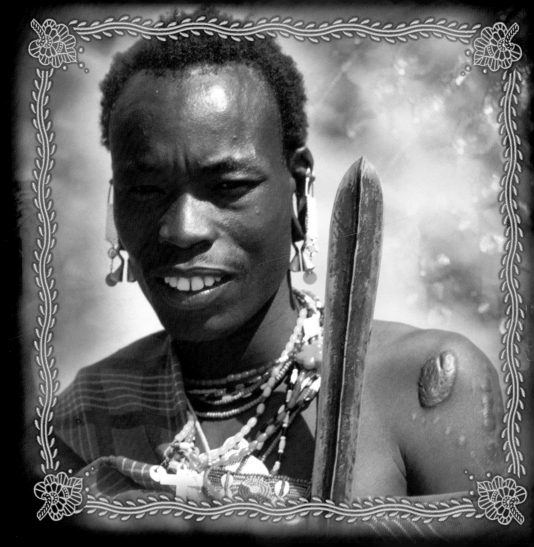

Scarification

One of the more extreme methods of body adornment is scarification. This is the process of the deliberate marking of the body with scars. The scars are often raised shapes, sometimes round or oval, which become part of the language inscribed on the body, each telling a story of pain, fortitude, sadness, or perhaps status. It has been practiced by many tribes throughout the world and examples can now be found in our modern society as a way of describing our own passage through life.

Papua New Guinea has an established ritual of scarification usually related to initiation of both men and women around the age of sixteen or seventeen. The cuts are usually made with a very sharp stone knife and are cauterized by a burning wand of a traditional medicine bush called a "conkerberry" which stops the bleeding. The stick remains on the cut until it has healed. Uninitiated people were banned from trading, getting married and singing ceremonial songs and today this still applies in some areas.

In the Sepik region, it is believed that the crocodile was the father of the human race. The return of the ancestral crocodile is celebrated during an initiation ceremony and cuts, which resemble crocodile teeth when healed, are made with a bamboo sliver on the chest, back and buttocks. The teeth-like scars represent the crocodile who has

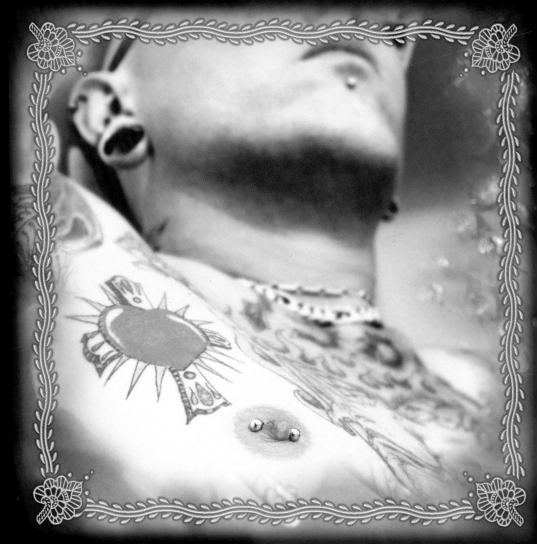

swallowed the initiates so that they can be reborn as crocodile-men. They bear their scars with pride, honoring a very special tradition of the people of Papua New Guinea.

Foot Binding

There are other ways to radically alter the actual shape of the body which may be pleasing to the cultural eye. Perhaps the most memorable is the crippling foot binding carried out for centuries on Chinese women. The practice began during the 10th century and was finally formally prohibited in 1911. It is thought that the practice has now died out, with the last factory which made shoes for bound feet closing in 1998. The agonizing process began when a child was five years old. Their feet were bound by their mothers and deliberately decreased in size over a period of months. The optimum length of a female foot was about three inches long—only then were the feet called "Lotus of Gold." Although feet became an object of devotion and admiration, women could only hobble and throughout their lives, their feet were a continual source of severe pain.

Head Reshaping

The head can be reshaped to great effect—the tribes of Vanautu prize an elongated head above all and respect its possessor as a person of great intelligence. It is known that some tribes began head

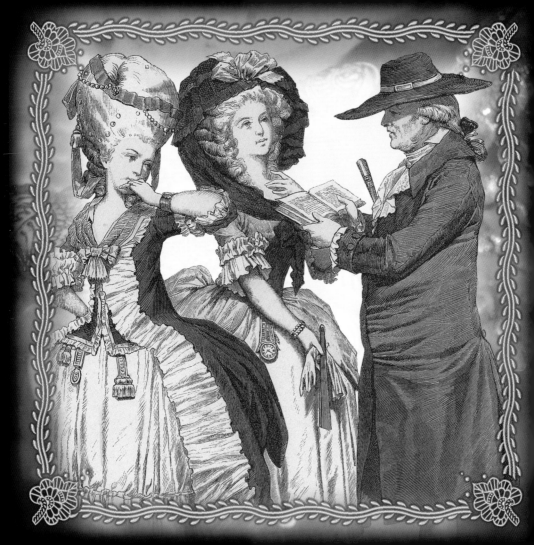

binding when a child was a month old and it normally took about six months for the required shape to develop. In the Congo, the Mangbetu people used cloth to bind babies' heads. In adulthood, the hair was wrapped around a basket frame to emphasize the elongated head. As late as the 19th century, head elongation was practiced in France and some other parts of Europe.

Different methods were used to encourage the reshaping, one being a tight bandage applied to a very young baby's head—as the child grew, the bandage was replaced with a rigid basket. The Bintulu Malanus Dayak people of Borneo considered a flat forehead a sign of beauty and also began the shaping process when the children were very young.

CORSETRY

Another example of body shaping is more Western in nature. Shaping the waist with whalebone corsetry tied with laces has its origins in the European Middle Ages. The corset was first worn outside the clothing. Victorian men and women popularized this way of hiding their bulges and emphasizing their straight backs. There are various modern types of underwear which are available to reshape bottoms and tummies, most of them just as uncomfortable and possibly not as effective!

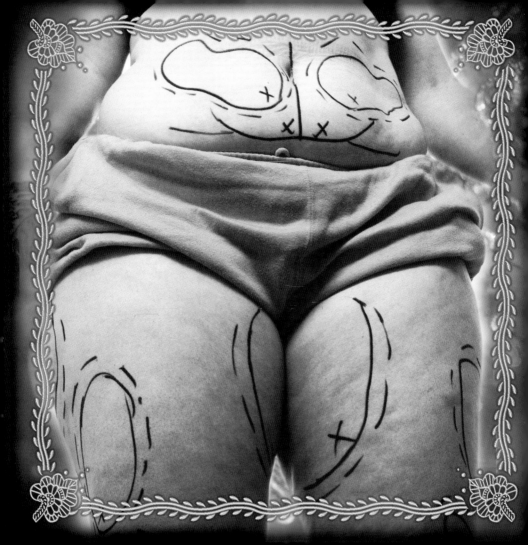

The Surgeon's Blade

The most popular form of body shaping today is cosmetic surgery. Practiced since at least 500 BC, cosmetic surgery is perhaps the ultimate ritual in body shaping—it is now possible to reshape or replace the entire exterior body. An action not to be taken lightly, for the consequences of cosmetic surgery can be severe if something goes wrong.

In our modern, disposable world, it seems not many of us are satisfied with our bodies. Some of us would change them in a heartbeat and go through anything to achieve the perfect look and body. Others of us go through the pain of scarification or body shaping as a rite of passage, a statement rejecting common values— our ancestors used body shaping and scarification to fit in with the demands of their society.

Some of us go through the same process to show our difference from everyone else.

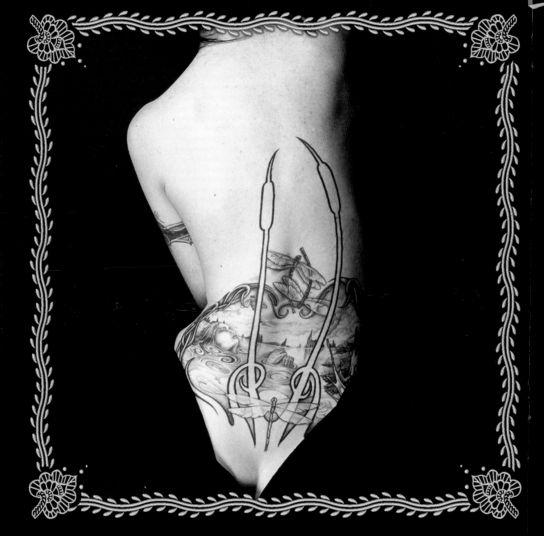

the art of TATTOO

The origin of the modern word "tattoo"
is said to have come from the Tahitian word
"tatu" or the Inuit word "tau-tau"—
both loosely meaning "to tap", the sound made by
banging one piece of sharp bone with
another to mark the skin.
Tattoos are made on the body by cutting or
pricking the skin and inserting pigment,
or coloring, into the scratch.

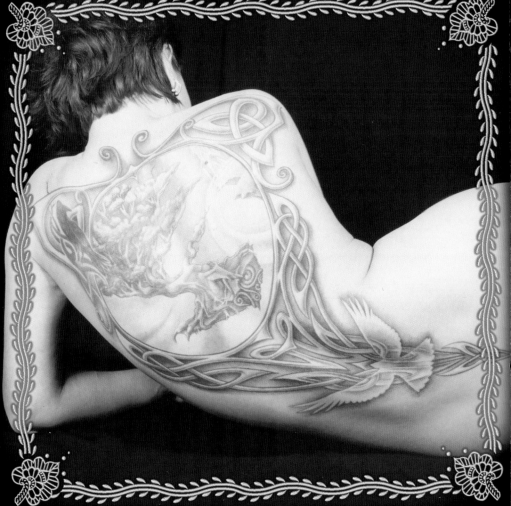

As the color is added under the skin, a tattoo is usually permanent. Devices used to prick the skin have included sharpened bones, thorns, knives, and needles but, today, most tattoos are done with an electric tattoo machine first invented in New York in 1891.

Many ancient cultures wore tattoos, including the Incas, Mayans, Aztecs, Greeks, Romans, and Egyptians—the purpose of tattooing varying from culture to culture. Staying healthy, warding off evil spirits, denoting social status or membership of a clan are just a few explanations of tattoo designs seen around the world.

Some nations have used tattoos in a more disturbing way—marking people as deserters, convicts and concentration camp prisoners to set them aside from others in the community. Even animals have tattoos inside their ears to identify them, and to ensure a safe return to their owners if they have strayed. Many tribes still continue to wear tattoos as a rite of passage and recognition within their own clan.

In today's modern world, we wear our tattoos with pride, having carefully chosen the design and colors ourselves. People can be seen who are living paintings; covered with stunning artwork from head to foot.

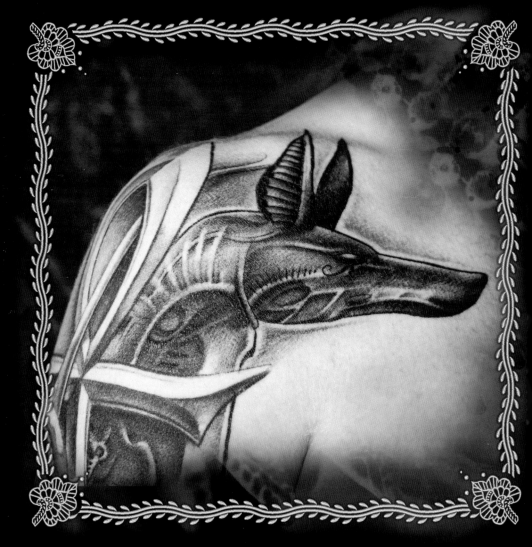

The Iceman

As one of the oldest forms of body art, marking our skin with tattoos is an enduring example of the human desire to decorate and adorn ourselves. The remarkable archaeological finds of recent years have confirmed the existence of tattoos centuries ago. One recent example is the discovery of "The Iceman," nicknamed Ötzi after the tztal Alps on the Austrian-Italian border where he was found in 1991. Apparently between 25 and 35 years old and suffering from arthritis when he died, his body has been carbon dated to 3300 BC. He has 57 tattooed marks, lines and dots on his back and legs, many of them located at acupuncture sites used today to treat arthritis.

Ritual Tattoos

Many ancient cultures used tattooing as part of their rituals. In recorded history, although it undoubtedly began earlier, Egyptian tattooing was first seen during the construction of the pyramids. The tattooed mummy of Amunet, a priestess of Hathor the Goddess of Love, was found at Thebes and is at least 4,000 years old. The tattoos located on the mummy's abdomen are presumably linked to fertility. A royal Egyptian child, dated from the same period, had the image of a sun god pricked into his skin, apparently by a bone needle; animal fat mixed with soot would have been the likely pigment.

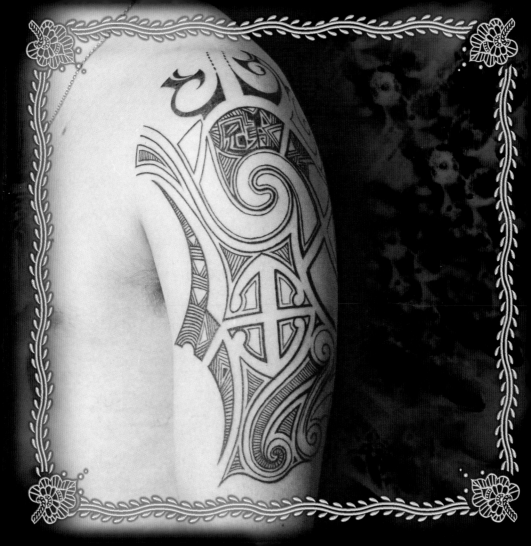

The Spread of Tattooing

The evidence uncovered thus far has helped us to trace the spread of tattooing around the world. As the Egyptian empire expanded, it is thought that the art became known in places like Greece, Persia, Central Asia and Arabia and along main merchant routes. Migrating southwards, tattooing spread to the Philippines, Borneo and the Pacific Islands, New Zealand and Polynesia.

Dating from around 2,400 years ago, at least two Pazyryk mummies have been found in the High Altai Mountains of western and southern Siberia. Their bodies were tattooed with a variety of animals including griffins and monsters, thought to be of magical significance. The Ancient Greeks learned tattooing from the Persians and the Romans from the Greeks. Mentioned in accounts by Plato, Aristophanes, Julius Caesar, and Herodotus, tattoos were generally used to mark slaves and punish criminals.

Not to be outdone, the Vikings tattooed family crests and tribal symbols on their bodies—still practiced today by some of their descendants. The early Celt tribes used tribal tattoos to intimidate and scare their enemy—Julius Caesar wrote about the terror inspired by their outlandish appearance. However, in the 4th century, the first

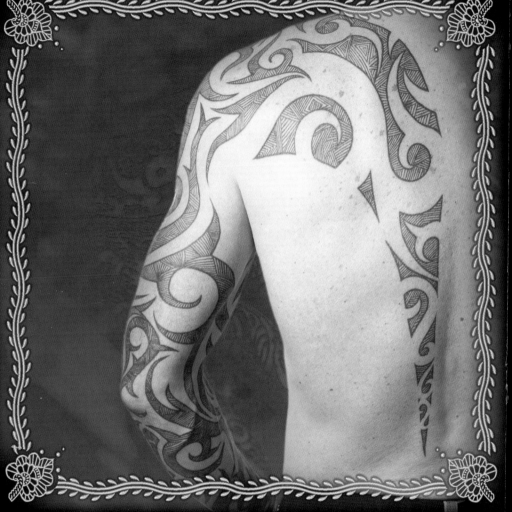

Christian emperor of Rome banned the tattooing of slaves and prisoners and in 787 AD, Pope Hadrian prohibited the practice altogether, although it still thrived in Britain until the Norman invasion of 1066. For around 500 years, tattooing was almost unknown in the Western world but continued unabated in the undiscovered places of the globe.

Tattoos have been used to teach, to scare, to shock, to identify, and to beautify, the human form. Although similar designs and symbols have been found in ancient examples of tattooing, their meanings differ from culture to culture. Much understanding of traditional tattooing has blurred with time, but it is recognized that many of today's patterns have their origins in the past, providing us with a rich insight into our heritage.

Samoan Tattoos

One island famous for its long history of tattooing is Samoa. The Samoan word "ta tau" (tattoo) means "appropriate, balanced and fitting." A form of fashion, for both men and women, a tattoo was also a statement of courage and ability to bear pain. Those who chose not to be tattooed were the subject of much condemnation by the other tribe members, but their reluctance is understandable when you consider that the common form of tattooing covered the entire lower body and could take as long as six months to finish!

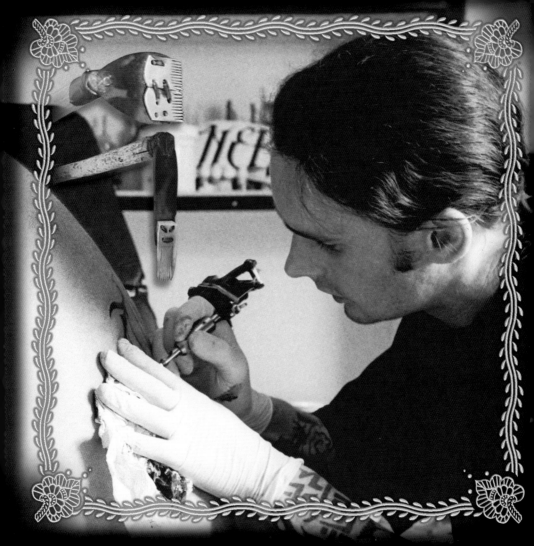

As with many cultures, tattooing was carried out in ritualistic fashion with a special hut being constructed for the process. Bone combs, first dipped in ink, were used to apply the design by tapping along the skin. Once the tattoo was complete, the hut was burnt down, marking progression into adulthood.

The word for a male tattoo was "pe'a," which means "flying fox," and refers to the dark charcoal color of the tattoo. The tattoo covers the area from knee to waist, each being completely unique but with recurring designs. The tattoo was always started in the small of the back (where the mythical figures of Taema and Tilafaiga were joined). The final design, the "pute," was drawn on the navel. Without this, the tattoo was considered unfinished and the wearer was forever shamed for not completing the ceremony.

A female tattoo was called "malu," which means to be protected and sheltered. As with the male tattoos, many designs were used, mostly for purely ornamental reasons, but an important recurring theme was a diamond shaped design on the back of the knee, also known as "malu."

How Ta Tau came to Samoa

A mythological fable about the origins of Samoan tattooing, this is the story of Taema and Tilafaiga who were Siamese twins joined at the spine, and were separated by a canoe while they were swimming. They traveled to the island of Fiji, where they were taught the art of tattooing by a pair of Fijian tattoo artists. When they returned to Samoa, Taema became a famous tattooist and teacher of the art and her sister, Tilafaiga, became a war goddess!

Other Traditions in the Pacific

The traditional tattoo technique and tools were much the same throughout most of the pacific islands. The designs, social significance, and position on the body differed greatly.

The Solomon Islands had a strong tradition of tattooing, which was carried out to the rhythmic beat of drums. A trance-like state normally resulted from the noise, providing relief from the pain. The more a man was tattooed, the greater his social standing became. It is said that this ethnic tradition died virtually overnight, with the complete conversion of the tribe by Seventh Day Adventists.

European explorers and the arrival of missionaries put a stop to the age-old tradition of tattooing in Tonga. Most Tongan men would have worn tattoos very similar to the Samoan traditional style. Women were also allowed to have tattoos as well but only on their arms and inside the hand. Tonga is unusual in that it has always retained its independence. However, with the mass acceptance of Christianity, many aspects of their ancient culture have been lost forever.

Tattooing was completely banned in 1838, and sadly both the art and the two thousand years of knowledge have almost disappeared. What is known is that a sharpened comb, made of bone or shell, was driven into the skin and a mixture of soot and water or fat was applied as the pigment.

Knowledge of traditional Tahitian tattooing is limited as well, but it was a "tapu" or "sacred" art form performed by highly trained professionals. The tool was similar to that used by the Tongans—a comb made of bone or shell with many needles secured onto a wooden shaft. The pigment used is made from soot mixed with water or oil and then pushed into the skin by the comb being tapped by a mallet-type implement.

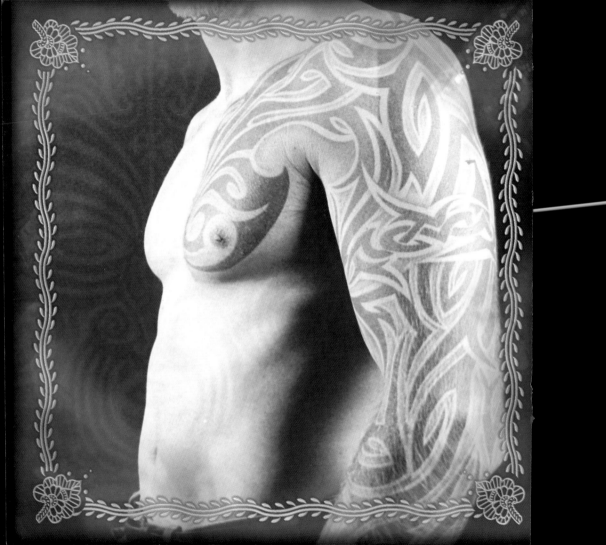

As with other cultures, the social implications of tattooing were immense. It could indicate sexual maturity, personal achievements and position in society. Almost everyone was tattooed in one form or another, that is until the arrival of missionaries, who banned the practice, seeing it as sinful. However, the art of tattooing is experiencing a resurgence of popularity as Polynesians rediscover their pride in their cultural heritage.

THE TA MOKO OF THE MAORIS

Probably the most famous tribal tattoo is the "Ta Moko" created by the Maoris of New Zealand. Worn by both men and women as a special honor, the designs are a living history of personal achievement and status within the tribe.

Only men were allowed a facial "moko" and no two faces were ever the same. The tattoo artist, also usually male, would study the face of his subject carefully. Each design was placed to accentuate individual facial features and was initially drawn with charcoal—the left side to show the father's history and the right side to tell the mother's history. Spirals and lines were drawn all over the face and then, using a very sharp bone or chisel, the artist would cut into the face. A pigment was made from burnt vegetables, caterpillars, or kapara tree bark, the soot then being mixed with oil or water in prized pots handed down through families. Indigo-black or blackish-green paste was then pressed into the cuts—a very painful procedure which caused swelling. It was forbidden to see a "Ta Moko" before it was finished.

Maori women were allowed to be tattooed on their chins, lips and shoulders while men often wore extensive body tattoos. Red, blue and black could be used for these less important markings. A special comb, with a wooden handle and several chisels, was used to tattoo large areas, including the buttocks, thighs, and genitals. Normally, swirling spirals, seen throughout the oceanic cultures, were drawn on the buttocks, the double spiral being commonly associated with the Maoris. Angular designs were drawn on the thighs and upper legs.

A rather ghastly trade ensued once explorers had seen the intricate designs on Maori heads. Preserved tattooed heads became a prized possession and were traded freely in Britain. This trade was finally outlawed in England in the 1830s but many heads remain in museums and collections today, despite Maori attempts to bring them home.

The legendary "Ta Moko" designs
of the Maori tribe are famous
all over the world today and re-created regularly
by modern tattoo artists.

How "Ta Moko" came to the Maoris

One day, visitors from the underworld, "Rarohenga," came to visit a Maori chief, Mataora. Mataora fell in love with one of them, Niwareka, who was the daughter of the underworld ruler, Vetonga. They were happily married for some years until Mataora became jealous and struck Niwareka. She fled home to her father and, desperately sorry and anxious to win her back, Mataora followed her and begged her forgiveness. He was kept away from her but her father agreed to tattoo his face. As he was being tattooed, he sang emotionally of his sorrow and his search for his wife. When she heard his words, Niwareka forgave him and they were allowed to return to "the upper world." The tattoo he bore on his face served as a reminder to avoid evil actions and so, the story goes, he introduced the art of tattooing to the upper world.

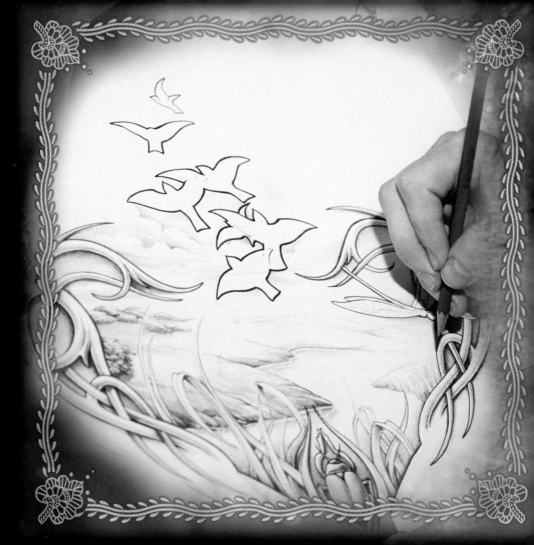

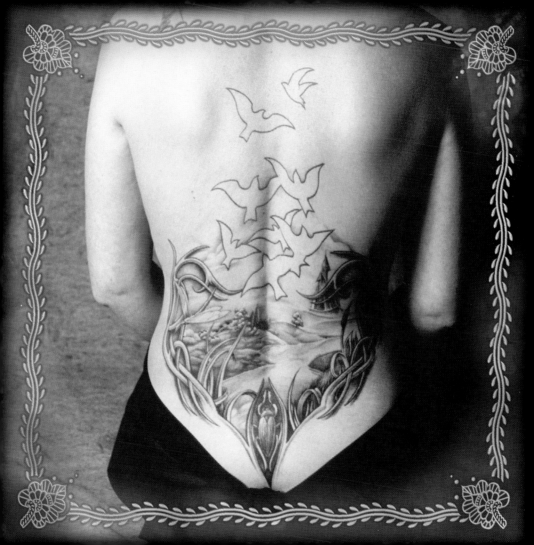

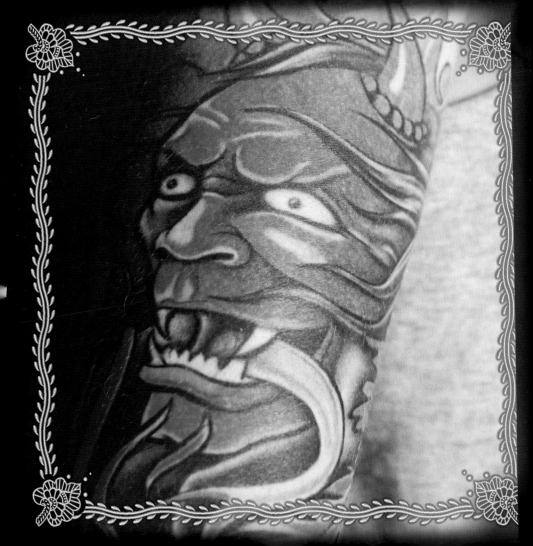

Japanese Tattoo

The art of tattooing has developed and flourished in Japan for centuries. Clay figures with facial masks, called "dogu" and dating back to at least 5000 BC have been unearthed in Japan. The markings on the mouths of the dogu resemble the tattoos decorating the mouths of women from the Ainu, who apparently took tattooing culture with them when they crossed over to the Japanese islands.

Recorded by Chinese historians in the 3rd century, the men of "Wa" (Japan) wore painted designs on their bodies and tattoos on their faces.

A later history, written in 622 AD, discusses the tattooing rituals of the Ryukyu Islands, where women, and sometimes men, were tattooed all over the back of their hands, and up to their elbows in some cases.

The symbolic tattooing of the tribe was an indication of marriage status and tribal customs, sometimes displaying their religious beliefs and sexual maturity.

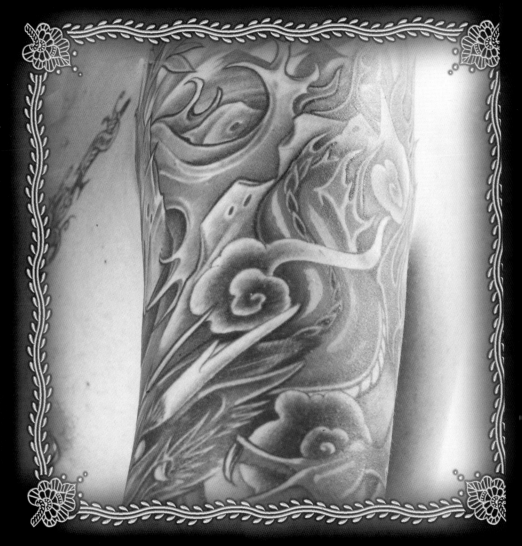

In the 15th century, an explorer discovered that the Ainu tribe wore many tattoos on their faces and the backs of their hands and arms. To enhance their appearance, women were tattooed around the lips, cheeks, forehead, and sometimes the eyebrows.

Traditionally, mothers created moustaches for their daughters by making small knife cuts on the upper lip and rubbing soot in the wounds. The first incision was made when the child was about two, and new ones were added every year until the girl was married.

At one time the women wore chastity belts and it was noted that the tattoo patterns on their bodies are quite similar in design and possibly symbolize virtue. Both the Ainu and people of the Ryukyu tribes believed that tattoos had healing properties when applied to the site of ill-health.

Traditional Japanese tattoos are known as "horimono"—"hor" or "horu" meaning "to carve" and "mono" meaning "thing." Carving is an excellent way of describing the methods used by 19th-century tattoo artists to perform their work. Sharp needles tied to a long bamboo handle were used to insert ink into the skin, although this is apparently a lot less painful than our Western methods. This elaborate pictorial fashion was first started by firemen, rickshaw drivers and others, who, because of their lowly station in life, were forbidden to wear the fine clothing of the upper classes and thus chose their own form of decoration.

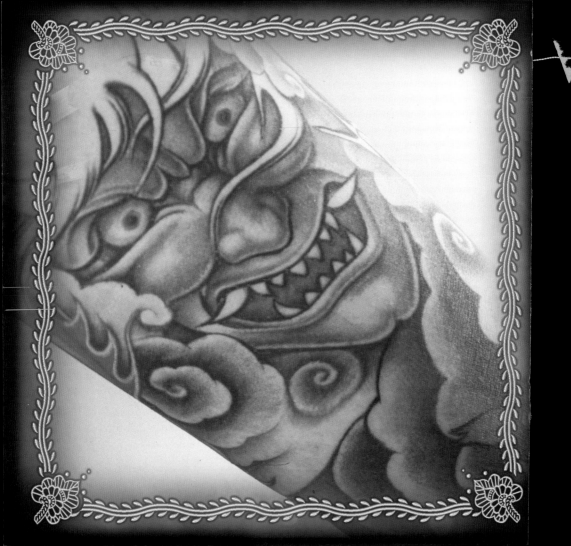

The art form, which developed from these humble beginnings, is both visually stunning and an extremely complex, tattooing style. Traditional Japanese tattoo artists will choose your design for you, and although the outer design may be traced by a modern, electric machine, the shading and color will almost certainly be completed in the horimono custom.

"Horimono" tattoos attribute their great beauty to the "ukiyoe" art upon which they are based, particularly that of master artist Utagawa Kuniyoshi. They are symbolic of a uniquely Japanese tradition of using designs handed down for centuries, preserving a rich and long cultural history.

Tattooing in the Americas

The Mayans and other South American tribes had been practicing the art since at least the 12th century and probably much before that. The belief that tattoos symbolized courage and bravery was strong, but conversely, tattoos were also used to mark the heads of criminals so all would know of their crimes.

There was a widespread practice of tattooing among Native Americans but unfortunately it is not very well documented.

What is known is that each tribe had its unique approach to tattooing customs and rites. Tattoos could symbolize adulthood, spiritual guides and achievement in battle. Quite often, a skilled person could be recognized by their tattoo and certainly tribes were identified by their markings.

Men and women were commonly tattooed among the Miami, Delaware and Winnebago tribes and the Houma tribe tattooed extensively on the body and the face. The Chickasaw men removed all their hair for large body coverage and outstanding warriors were recognized by their tattoos. Other tribes, such as the Chitimacha and Acolapissa, wore very little clothing to display the extensive artwork on their bodies.

The Ojibwa tattooed the temples, forehead and cheeks of headache sufferers in a ceremony to ward off evil spirits and hopefully cure the headache! Interestingly, it is said that the Inuit women had their chins tattooed as a fertility charm. During puberty, they were tattooed on their chins, nose, cheeks, legs, and arms— endurance of the pain was considered proof that a woman was ready for childbirth.

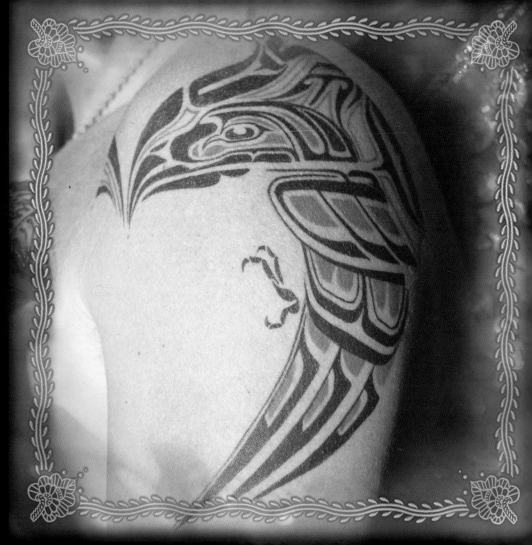

The Impact of Missionaries

Jesuit missionaries, mainly based in eastern Canada, sent regular reports back to their countries during their travels in North America and were horrified by the tattooing practices they witnessed. The common practice of piercing the skin with a thorn and pasting berry juice or soot into the wound was considered dangerous and barbaric. Thought of as the work of Satan, the tattoos exhibited spiritual and magical images. Once the Americas had been colonized, many tribal customs were considered unacceptable and tattoos were rarely seen on Native American people.

There's no Business like Show Business

In the 1800s, the bizarre entertainment of tattoo exhibitions was brought to the general public with tattoo circuses using live subjects. It quickly became widespread in the United States. The first man to be exhibited was thought to be James F O'Connel who was employed by PT Barnum's Museum. His extensive tattoos had been forcibly applied, or so he said, while in captivity on a South Sea island. Once the tattoo machine was developed, fully tattooed people began appearing in circuses and sideshows. Tattoo artists would travel with the circus, ready to practice their art on eager customers. In 1871, the first traveling tattooed man in America was a Greek

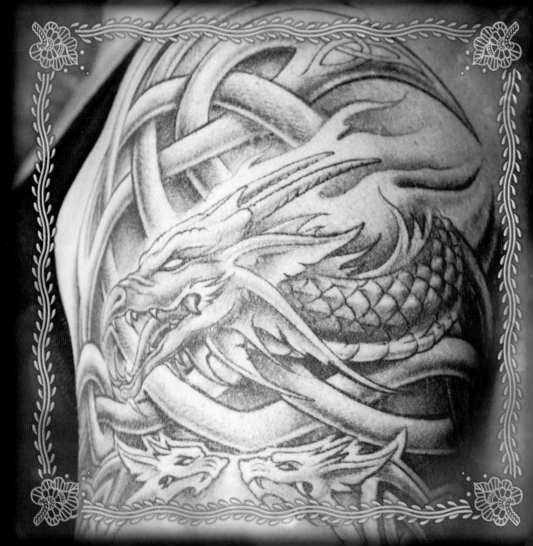

called Constantine, who also claimed he had been tattooed by force while in captivity but in reality was tattooed in Burma. He had 388 elaborate tattoos which ensured a very successful show business career.

As with many other people of the world, many Americans are now reviving their traditional heritage by using the old tribal tattoo designs.

Western Europe and Britain

Tattooing in Western Europe and Britain certainly has a long, if interrupted, history. Pre-Celtic Iberians in the British Isles were tattooed in special ceremonies, as were the Gauls and many of the Teutonic tribes, while the Danes, Norsemen and Saxons wore family symbols and crests on their chests. As we would see later, Christian civilization did much to dispel the traditions of European tattooing. In 787 AD the Pope banned the practice, allowing only criminals to be branded. Solely in Britain did some traditions manage to survive.

Tattooing flourished in Britain until the Norman Invasion of 1066. King Harold, killed in battle at Hastings, was only identified by the word "Elizabeth" which he had tattooed over his heart. The Normans disapproved heartily of tattooing and there is little mention of it in British records from the 12th to the 16th centuries, although during the Crusades, the crusaders tattooed a cross on their arms to ensure a Christian burial if they died in foreign lands.

Conquest and Discovery

As Europe conquered the world and discovered unknown countries with their many pagan and savage practices, the lost art of tattooing became better known again.

In the 16th century, Sir Martin Frobisher set off on a voyage to find the northwest passage to China. Although he failed in his quest, he apparently returned to England with an Inuit woman who had traditional tattooing on her forehead and chin. Stories of tattooed people had been told for many years by sailors returning from their travels so actually witnessing tattoos caused quite a stir in England.

It wasn't long before seamen from all over Europe began returning home with tattoos all over their own bodies. It rapidly became quite a tradition with the British Royal Navy, although the French navy and army banned tattooing within their ranks.

In the 18th century, the famous Captain Cook, using the word "tattaw" to describe a tattoo, studied the Tahitian way of tattooing, making notes of the designs and tools used, and eventually being tattooed himself. Sydney Parkinson, who traveled with him as expedition artist, created a pictorial record, which can still be seen today, of some of the most fascinating designs of the Pacific Islands.

The sailors who traveled with the expeditions were astonished by the painful process and the end result and spread the word at home. Similar events occurred throughout Europe, the Western world gradually being reintroduced to this once "sinful" artform.

For a short time, tattoos became popular among the upper classes in England. In 1862, the Prince of Wales received the first of many tattoos—a Jerusalem cross—after visiting the Holy Land. Twenty years later, his sons, the Duke of Clarence and the Duke of York (later King George V) had dragons tattooed on their arms by the Japanese master tattooist, Hori Chiyo.

Tattooing in the Modern World

Tattooing in Europe today is much the same as elsewhere. Modern technology ensures a lower health risk and many designs are freely available. Increasingly, people are searching the past for designs and we are, in the process, reviving old customs.

Tattooing is enjoying a new lease of life in recent times. Considered to be dangerous, unhygienic and socially unacceptable for many years, the attitude towards body marking has undergone a great change. The safer methods now used and the large availability of tattoo artists and designs have all contributed to the successful reintroduction of tattooing.

Television programs, books, and magazines about tattoos are readily available for the tattoo enthusiast to follow the latest fashion. The internet has spawned many sites which advertise tattoo artists and showcase their work, along with many designs and general information about tattooing. Strict regulations ensure that most tattoo parlors, and their artists, are properly equipped and trained, and no longer found in the less salubrious areas of town.

A trend towards the bizarre was once quite common throughout the United States and England. Freak shows have also regained popularity and an example of this is the Jim Rose Circus which exhibits many strange and gruesome acts, including a man transformed into a lizard by tattooing and body modification.

Tattoo conventions have become regular events, where the extremes of body modification and tattooing are on display. People come to display their own tattoos and can have new ones added. New designs and old mingle here, with the common thread of the love of tattoos pulling everyone together.

Once seen as bizarre
and non-Christian,
tattoos have become more acceptable as we
discover their origins and
tribal importance.

Many different cultures and their tattoo patterns have been discussed in this book. The desire to return to historical roots has led to a strong revival of traditional ethnic tattooing—witness the resurgence of the "Ta Moko" originally worn by the fearsome Maori warriors and now commonplace at tattoo conventions. The traditional Japanese and Celtic designs are just as popular and even old sailor designs are reappearing on modern skin.

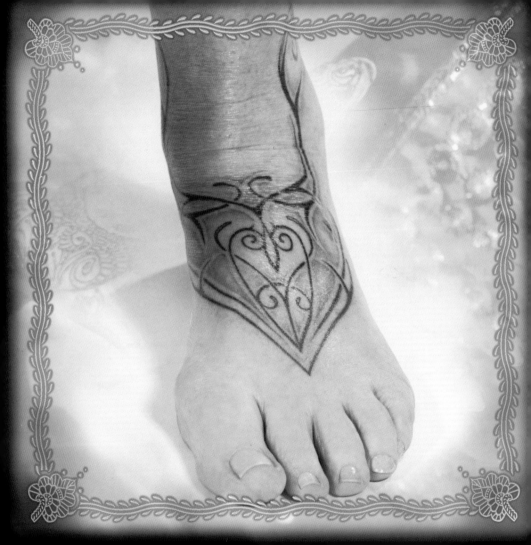

The nature of modern society has dictated that "we want what we want now" and every facet of our lives is geared to this premise. The nature of tattooing, however, prevents instant gratification—a reputable artist must be found, an appointment made, a design chosen. Time is needed to complete the work and a period of healing required before a tattoo can be fully enjoyed.

Whether you choose to have a simple tattoo, on an undisclosed location on your body, or a huge dragon on your face, the world still has a long way to go before every possible tattoo design has been drawn on the human form. We like to think we are unique, but as we have seen, time and time again, all the body art discussed in this book has evolved from common ancient roots. Certainly older than most present cultural practices, tattooing is now an individual craft performed mainly for individual reasons but mainly for self-adornment.

A Note About Safety
The dangers of having a tattoo need to be considered seriously. Any invasive procedure on the body carries a risk of infection, and it is wise to consider all the facts before you decide to go ahead.

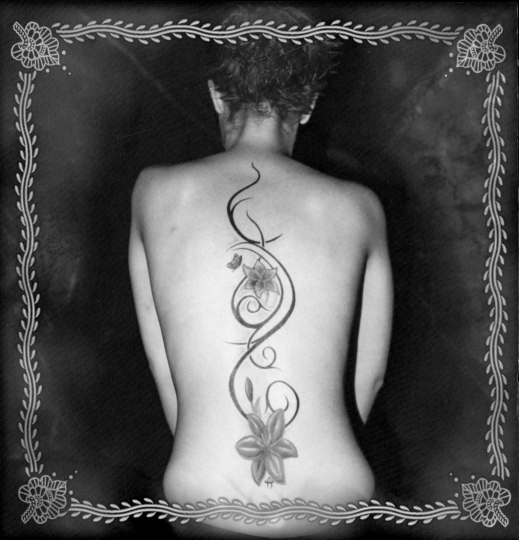

A doctor should be consulted, if you have any illnesses such as diabetes, hepatitis or any other blood-borne disease, before you have a tattoo. If you are taking any blood-thinning drugs, such as aspirin, or have a disorder that causes you to bleed more than usual, having a tattoo can be an unnecessary risk to your health.

People have experienced various allergic reactions during, and after, being tattooed. Fortunately this is rare and there are remedies available, which will help. Some individuals have a high degree of reaction to foreign material and the process of tattooing can trigger lumps and itching.

Once you have decided to go ahead, find a reputable tattoo artist who comes well recommended. When you make the initial appointment, you should ask about all the training they have had and if there are any certificates available to verify this. You need to ensure that they disinfect any needles in an autoclave, which is a sterilizing unit capable of killing every living microorganism. A professional will always wear gloves and should remove new sterile needles from an autoclave bag in front of you and dispose of them safely afterward. Most countries impose an age restriction of eighteen years or older.

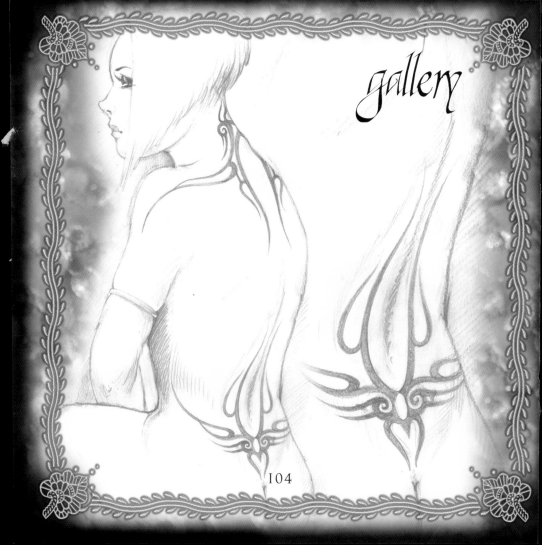

gallery

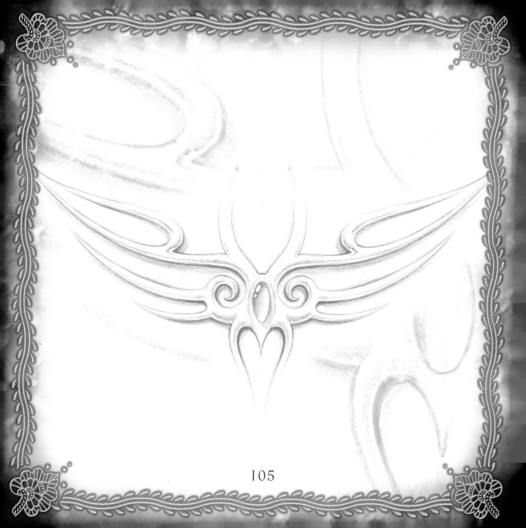

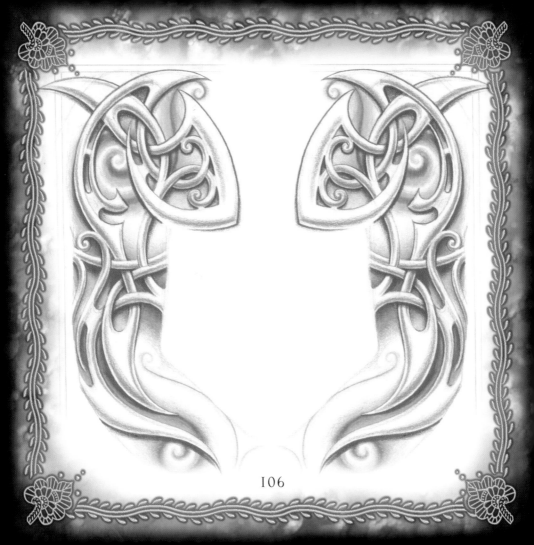

106

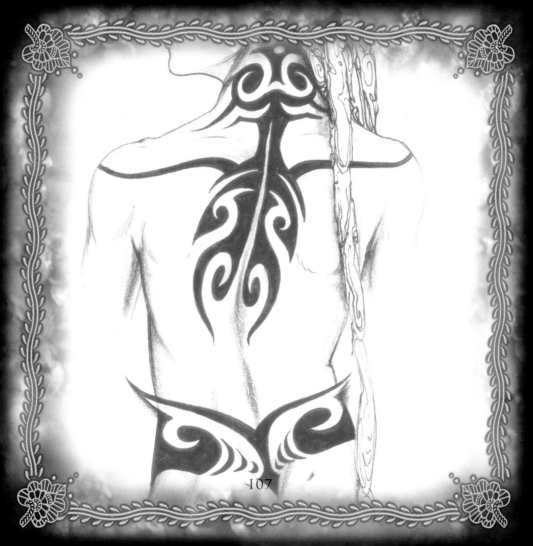

108

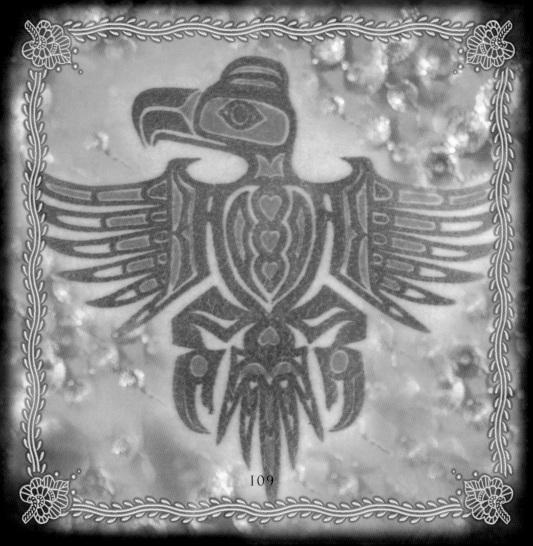

109

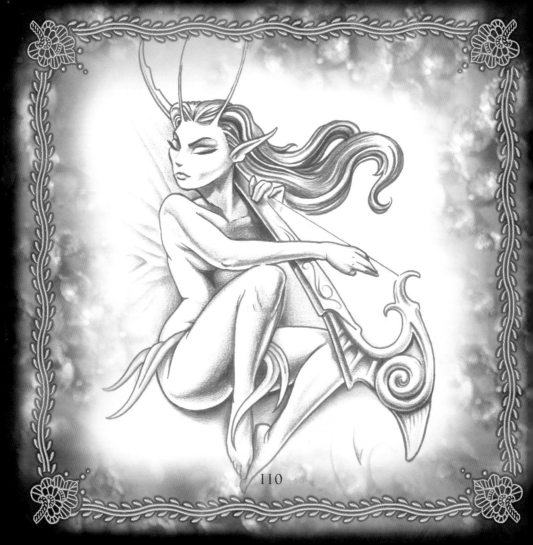

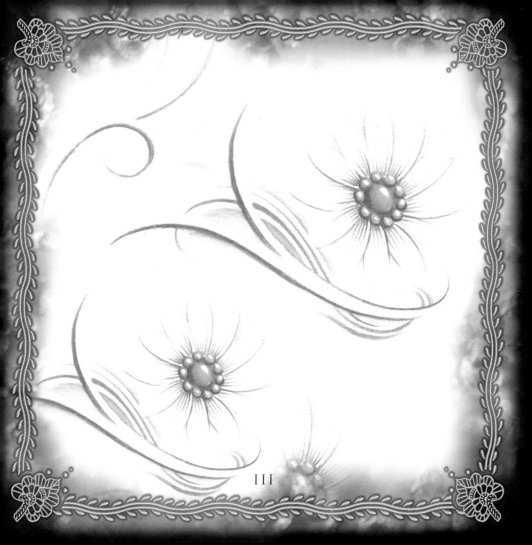

III

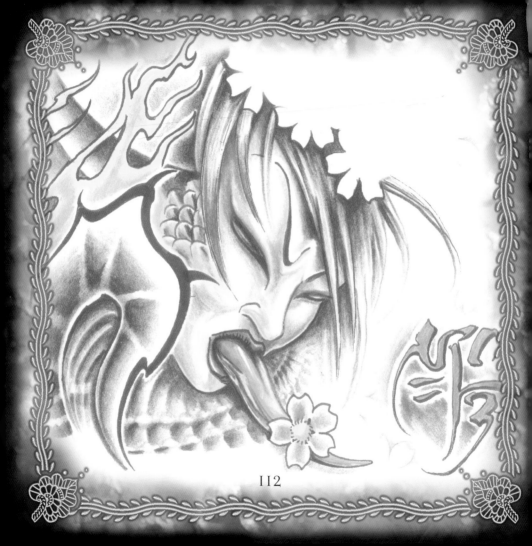

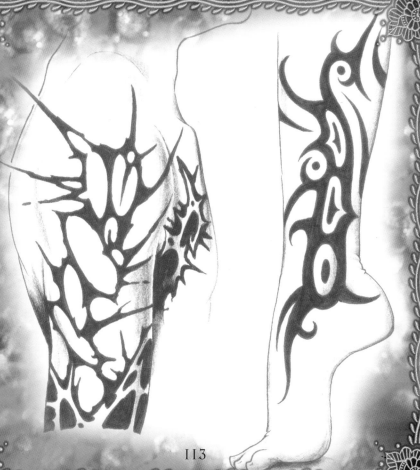

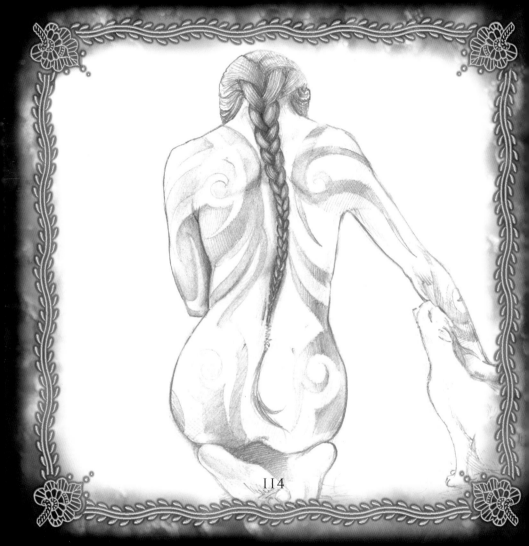

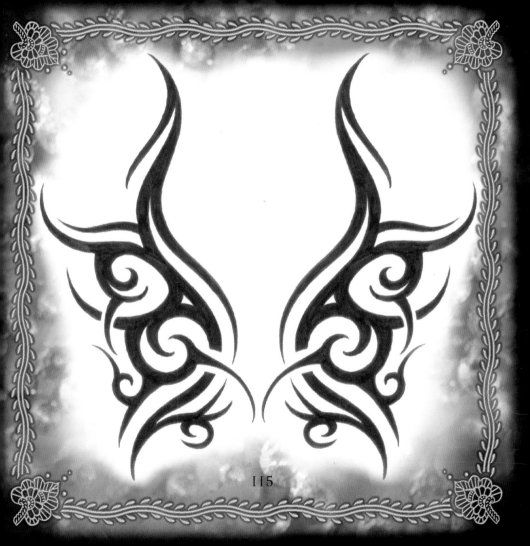

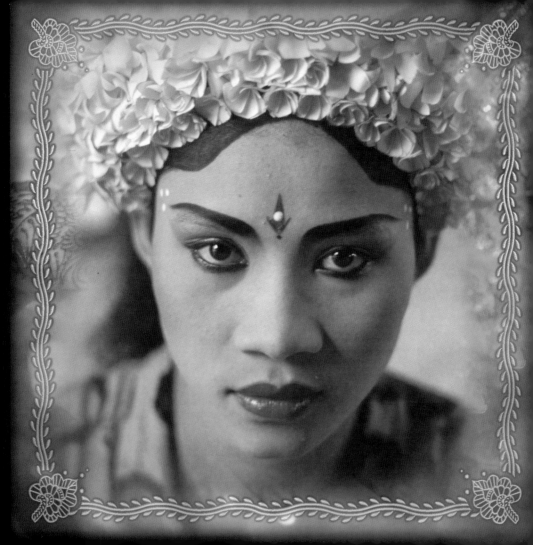

ACCESSORIES *body*

Throughout our existence,
the human race has always sought to change our
outward appearance by either altering
the body itself or decorating it.
Natural objects, such as seeds, grass, shells,
stones, wood, and feathers,
have all been used to enhance appearance.

The first jewelry of civilization was probably purely for self-expression, but the need for personal talismans followed quickly, many ornaments being worn to protect the body from evil spirits and bad luck! There are old paintings and sculptures which confirm how common the practice was. Early humans were very creative, given that they had no technology and few of today's benefits at hand.

Hawaiian Leis

The island cultures had access to wonderful shells and it is recorded that the first use of cowrie shells for body adornment was 8000 BC. There is no date provided for the origination of the craft of Hawaiian lei-making, but the placing of a sweet-smelling garland of flowers around a visitor's neck has provided many memorable arrivals to the islands. Made from flowers, ferns, herbs, nuts, seeds, pods, shells, and feathers, the lei can be worn around the neck or the head, around the wrist or ankle, or draped over the arm. Fresh leis, made of leaves and flowers, are most frequently made to mark a special occasion, particularly rites of passage such as marriage, departure or death.

Indian Jewelry

The familiar sight of gold jewelry on beautiful Indian women has been the envy of many. Exquisitely crafted jewelry has a long tradition in India—one interesting item, the "kamarbandhs" is worn around the waist and was once used for checking any weight change by the queen.

The Naga tribes of northeast India have a ceremonial ritual dress, decorated with the feathers of a hornbill and worn only by those of a high status. The tusk of a boar, worn as a necklace or through the earlobe, is considered to be the insignia of a warrior.

Many other natural materials are used for their body adornment, such as teeth, shells, and wood. Often the items are passed down from parents to children and prized as family heirlooms but they can also be acquired as a reward for performing a brave act.

Ornaments are also used for the purpose of ethnic identification and throughout India, most tribes have very different reasons for wearing their specific jewelry. People believe that ornaments made of iron create magic and that wearing iron rings is a protection against lightning. Similarly, iron neckbands are used to ward off witchcraft and iron hairpins as a cure for a headache.

Aboriginal Adornments

Although best known for their ferocious body painting, ornaments were also worn by many Aboriginal groups. Desert women wore strings of red "ininti" beans diagonally across the chest and in other areas, animal teeth and bones were made into necklaces with bird feathers. In coastal areas, women made necklaces from shells collected on the seashore.

African Storytellers

African beadwork can be seen throughout Africa, a result of the early visits by explorers, who brought glass beads for trade. Best known of all, the Zulu people of KwaZulu, Natal, in South Africa, have a unique bead culture, weaving eloquent stories of love and pain into the patterns.

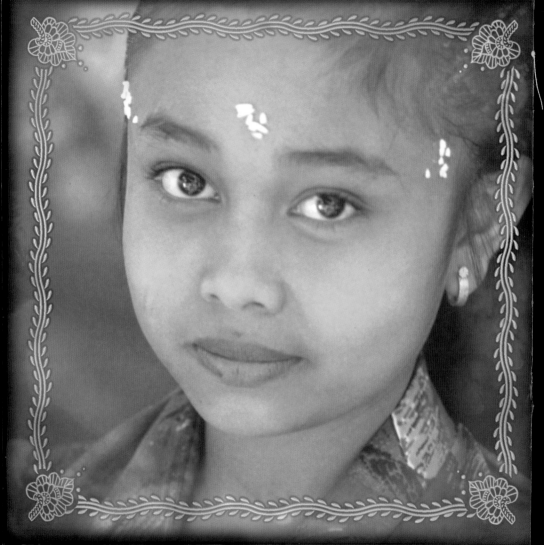

There are many more tribes who continue to wear traditional items as a signal of pride and honor. Our modern body adornment is an extension of old ideas and new technology—there is no sign that wearing items to enhance the appearance will ever fade from fashion.

Jewelry in the Modern World

There are many parts of the body which are enhanced by the use of jewelry. Almost everyone wears some form of jewelry, whether it is a chain, a ring, a bracelet, or earrings, and it has long been an acceptable form of self decoration. There are many items which both men and women can wear and the barriers between the sexes appear to be well and truly down.

If you like wearing jewelry, the choices are huge. One of the most innovative new arrivals on the jewelry scene is temporary body gems, now readily available, which can be attached to any part of the face or body to create a big impact. Temporary navel gem tattoos look very real when applied and can save you the pain and hassle of having your naval pierced. A nose piercing can be faked with the judicious placing of a tiny stud or gem. They are easy to remove and can sometimes be used again. As most reputable suppliers will have ensured that they are cosmetically safe, with the added advantage of a changed appearance each time a different gem is applied, there is no reason not to have a go!

Whether you choose gold or silver, beads or fake gemstones, jewelry is now widely available in any shape or form, to suit any budget. Obviously quality will differ between the more expensive and the cheaper lines, but the choice is certainly a far bigger one than was available to our ancestors.

Bindi and the Spiritual Third Eye

The mysterious and evocative bindi, worn as a badge of honor by many women, has a profound symbolism deep rooted in ancient folklore. The decorative mark signifies the mystic or spiritual third eye, "Ajana Chakra," and is positioned on the forehead between the eyes—traditionally the seat of latent wisdom and the place of the 6th Chakra, which governs brain activity If the bindi is properly marked, it becomes the central point at the base of creation itself, preserving power and energy within the body.

A symbol of good fortune, festivity and joy, the word bindi is derived from the Sanskrit word "bindu" meaning a drop or dot. The bindi is also referred to as a "tilak," "pottu" or "tikka" and has many other names. There are people who believe that applying the bindi with an ash paste signifies their humbleness, but to many the small red circle on a woman's forehead customarily indicates her married status—when in mourning or widowed, she will not wear one at all.

As part of the Hindu marriage ceremony, a dot of red kumkum, made from flower petals is pressed to her forehead and many associate this with the ancient practice of offering blood sacrifices to appease the gods.

There are many other traditional beliefs regarding the bindi. Shiva, the God of Destruction, destroys fire when he opens his third eye located on his forehead. It is believed that the placing of the bindi on their own third eye will protect humans and calm them when angry. Both men and women wear bindi to give themselves peace of mind—Hindu men using an elongated shape instead of the dot.

The traditional red powder applied to the forehead is bright red mercuric sulfide, vermilion. Other powders used are made from turmeric and alum, and sometimes ashes, sandalwood and turmeric. Fashion stakes today have ensured that the bindi is available for all to wear in many flamboyant colors and styles, sticky-backed gems and felt shapes. The special feeling of becoming a part of a very special sisterhood is created when the bindi is placed on your forehead.

Bindi Designs
When positioning a single bindi on your forehead, ensure that it is centered between the eyebrows and slightly above the brow line.

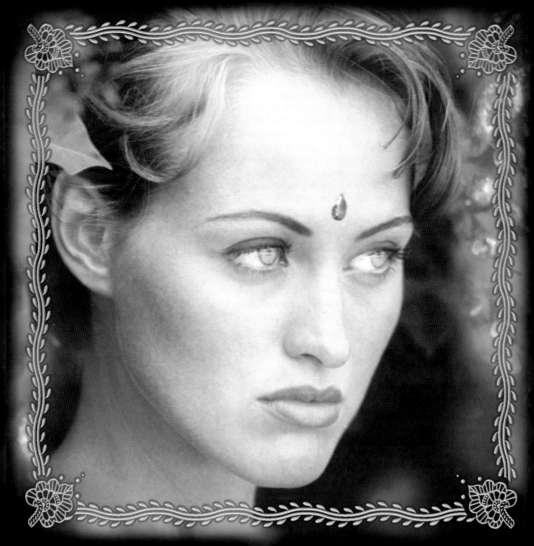

Here are a few suggestions for applying temporary gems, which are readily available from many street stores. Always perform a patch test before using a new supply of body gems.

A Grand Night Out

Wearing a single clear crystal bindi teardrop supplied with this pack, can be a very striking way of showing off your face and enhancing your special outfit. When placing the bindi, ensure that the narrowest part of the decoration points towards your hairline.

A Special Event

Using a teardrop-shaped bindi, place centrally between the eyebrows, with the narrowest part pointing upwards. Add the small circles outwards from the central bindi, following the arch of the eyebrows.

Red Sunset

For this design, you will need a large, red, double-beaded body gem and some smaller red gems. Place the large gem in the correct bindi position. Place a small bindi on either side of the central point of the double beaded gem. Then, radiating outwards, add more gems on either side.

Traditional

Place a single spot or circular gem between your eyebrows, and secure it in the bindi position.

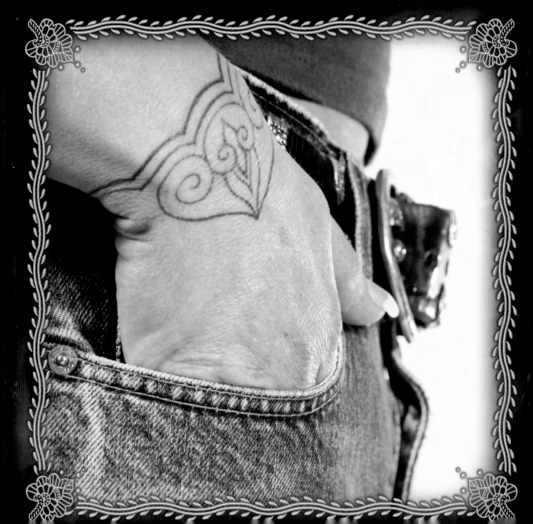

CONCLUSION

Body art has undergone a huge revival in recent years.

It serves as a tool for self expression as well as a means of re-creating the traditions of the past.

Modern methods still mirror the original ways used to perform body art, and quite a lot of ancient designs and ideas have been recovered and are now being used again.

Many people are searching for some form of identity and are using very different ways to find it. Tattoos and jewelry are worn to deliberately flout normal convention, the more bizarre and outrageous the better, as people try to imprint their bodies with a unique identity.

In most cases, we do not decorate our body for any deep or meaningful reason today although the trend towards discovering ourselves through the past continues.

Self-Decoration is a personal quest to attain that special look and thankfully we all have different ideas of the perfect appearance.

As the art of painting and tattooing the body continues to develop, the road ahead is not clear. What else can be decorated and adorned on the human body? Has everything been tried? It seems unlikely, so long may the quest for perfection continue.

EXPLORE THE WORLD OF

BODY ART

AND BODY ADORNMENT

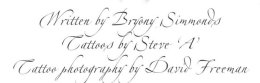

Written by Bryony Simmonds
Tattoos by Steve 'A'
Tattoo photography by David Freeman

TOP THAT!™

Copyright © 2004 Top That! Publishing plc,
Top That! Publishing, 25031 W. Avenue Stanford,
Suite #60, Valencia, CA 91355
All rights reserved
www.topthatpublishing.com

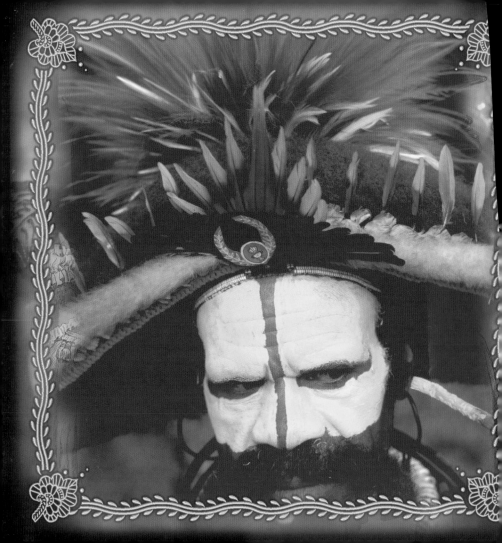